Brain Fog

Brain Fog

Solve the mysteries of decreased mental capacity and keep your brain fit and functional throughout your life

Binyamin Rothstein, D.O.

iUniverse, Inc.
New York Lincoln Shanghai

Brain Fog
Solve the mysteries of decreased mental capacity and keep your brain fit and
functional throughout your life

iUniverse books may be ordered through booksellers or by contacting:

iUniverse
2021 Pine Lake Road, Suite 100
Lincoln, NE 68512
www.iuniverse.com
1-800-Authors (1-800-288-4677)

The suggestions in this book are not meant to be a substitute for a careful
medical evaluation by your doctor. This book is intended for educational
purposes and the use of the information presented should be used with
discretion.

ISBN-13: 978-0-595-33894-8 (pbk)
ISBN-13: 978-0-595-78679-4 (ebk)
ISBN-10: 0-595-33894-1 (pbk)
ISBN-10: 0-595-78679-0 (ebk)

Printed in the United States of America

I dedicate this book to my wife Rivka and our children: Shlomo, Shaina, Sara Gita, Shmuel, Tsippi, Chaya Mushka, Menucha Bracha, and Eliana Simcha—you are my most precious gifts.

ACKNOWLEDGEMENTS

Brain Fog required the support and assistance of many people. Many thanks to Dr. Ronald Klatz, founder of the American Academy of Anti-Aging Medicine, and a long-time friend, who initiated the book concept when he asked me to present this topic at a Chicago conference in 2001. A big thank you to the library staff at the Sinai Hospital in Baltimore, Maryland, including Lee Cook, Lillian Himes, and Kay Wordlaw. Special Thanks to Mary Jo Fahey, who helped with the organization and publishing of the book. To my office staff, Shoshana Millstone and Rita Vitas—your patience and dedication do not go unnoticed. A special thank you also goes to Terri Lorden who patiently typed, retyped, retyped, and retyped—all with a smile.

To my parents Mr. Arnold Rothstein (o.b.m.), Mrs. Phyllis Rothstein (may she live and be well) and my mother-in-law Mrs. Anne Luborsky (o.b.m.), my heartfelt gratitude for all of your years of love and support.

My deepest unending appreciation goes to my wife, Rivka. In addition to making great chicken soup, she is a supportive, encouraging and tolerant wife. She transformed my "medicalese" into English, displaying great patience, diligence and dedication, not to mention talent and insight. Without Rivka's aid, this book could never have been completed.

Finally, I am grateful and humbled by the bountiful gifts and blessings bestowed upon me by the Al-mighty. His ways are just and His truth is eternal.

CONTENTS

CHAPTER 1

Introduction

The brain is the most amazing, magnificent and complex organ of your body. The human brain not only controls our instinctual survival mechanisms but allows us the expression of our highest selves—our ability to conceptualize, to choose between right and wrong, to dream, hope, pray and express ourselves to others in words.

The brain, however is still an organ of flesh and blood and therefore can be compromised by many different factors. Like a radio whose reception is full of static because certain components need to be cleaned and repaired, our brain's reception can also become "fuzzy" due to such simple factors as lack of sleep or poor diet to more complex reasons such as allergies, hormonal imbalances and toxins. This "fuzziness" which diminishes our ability to think clearly, to remember and communicate effortlessly is what we call "Brain Fog."

Living with brain fog means living suboptimally. We may survive but we don't thrive. We are less energetic and less enthusiastic. We are more easily frustrated and reactive and less proactive. Just getting through the day takes more effort as we try to function and focus through the "fog."

It wasn't until after I became a doctor and was doing research in a medical library that I started noticing in the literature all of the connections between brain function and such factors as toxins, food allergies, and hormones. I began to look at my own life and saw how my own functioning had been compromised by a number of the factors I will address in this book.

For instance, while growing up I had the standard dental care, which meant getting "silver fillings" whenever I had a cavity. By the time I was in junior high school my mouth was full of "silver fillings". Little did we suspect that these fillings were not silver at all but 50% mercury. Whoever dreamed that mercury, one of the most toxic metals on the planet, was being stuck in our teeth and that the effect of its toxic buildup could take years to show up and contribute to a decrease in brain function.

In high school I remember thinking "if I could just stay on track and keep a clear head and stay focused, I could do so much better in school." I was a good student and no one else could tell, but I knew I was working too hard to learn things. Could it have been the mercury in my "silver" fillings affecting my brain?

After starting my research, I decided to see for myself. I went to a dentist who specializes in removing mercury fillings and had my fillings replaced with composites. Within two days of having my fillings replaced, my Brain Fog worsened to such a degree that I struggled to continue my practice. Even though precautions had been taken, some mercury had escaped into my system during the removal. With enormous effort, I went back to researching how I could heal myself. Neither the dentist nor I had realized the need for mercury detoxification both before and after having the fillings removed. I started on a detoxification and vitamin regimen and not only did my Brain Fog completely clear, but I felt better than ever.

Food sensitivities and their association with Brain Fog became a reality to me when I was in the army. I was scheduled to see the deputy post commander right after my lunch break. For lunch I ate cheese and crackers. Soon after, my speech started to slur and I got so groggy I fell fast asleep (actually more like "passed out") right in the chair where I was sitting. I slept for over an hour and when I got up I felt foggy and fuzzy. I returned to the clinic to find out that a very angry deputy post commander had just left my office after having waited for over half an hour. In the army, one does not keep a full colonel waiting, especially when he's the deputy post commander.

I had never before noticed the correlation between what I ate and how I felt, but this episode made me realize that I have a food sensitivity to wheat and dairy. I now understood why, as a competitive tennis player in college, there were certain days I just felt too foggy, achy, stiff and unmotivated to compete. If only I had known then what I know now!

About ten years ago, while I was under an enormous amount of stress, I noticed a weakening of my mental processes. By then, my research had taught me that under stress, cortisol levels rise and in men, testosterone levels tend to decline. DHEA, a hormone critical for brain and immune function is also suppressed under great stress. I had myself tested, and sure enough, I was low in DHEA and testosterone. Once I began supplementing with DHEA and testosterone as well as taking 5HTP and pregnenolone to improve my sleep quality and protect my brain from excess cortisol, mental clarity and energy returned.

Like pieces of a puzzle that all began to fit together, I began to see how many different factors affected brain function in my patients. Hypothyroidism and the hormonal changes that come with PMS and menopause are strong factors that induce Brain Fog in women. Children and adults that have experienced injuries to the head and neck—even such innocuous events as accidental bumps—can experience symptoms of Brain Fog. Poor diet, hypoglycemia, metabolic deficiencies and infections have a significant role in Brain Fog.

How Do I Know If I Have Alzheimer's Dementia?

Of course, the most frequent question I am asked when people are frustrated and concerned by a lack of mental clarity is whether or not they are developing Alzheimer's Disease. We treasure our relationships, our independence, our growth, and above all, our dignity. No one wants to be placed in a nursing home bereft of respect and self-determination. In most cases, I can reassure them that they do not have Alzheimer's but are experiencing the effects of brain fog.

Alzheimer's Dementia (AD) is a progressive loss of memory that gradually begins to interfere with the activities of daily living. AD begins to change the brain by forming neurofibrillary tangles and senile plaques that contain A beta amyloid proteins. Usually the first indication that something is amiss is the inability to keep track of finances. People with AD may find themselves getting lost in what should be familiar territory. They begin misplacing objects and cannot find them, and familiar names and faces become unfamiliar. In addition to losing short-term memory, they also lose long-term memory. One of the diagnostic signs of AD is the inability to draw a clock showing 8:20. Yet, people with AD can maintain normal social graces, routine behavior, and superficial conversation. With the advent of sophisticated diagnostic equipment such as PET Scans, the diagnosis of AD is no longer confined to autopsy.

Progressive forgetfulness occurs in 10% of all people between the ages of 70 and 85. This means that 90% do not have Alzheimer's, although they may have some memory loss. Over age 85, 40% to 60% experience memory loss, but only 20%

to 30% actually have Alzheimer's. For those who have Alzheimer's, the chances of recovery are slim. The good news is that for the majority of people who are experiencing senile dementia (or forgetfulness), the problem may not be as difficult to treat as one may think. Once the cause of brain fog is narrowed down, a treatment plan can be outlined that will usually alleviate 80 to 90% of the symptoms and restore memory and brainpower.

Can Children Experience Brain Fog?

Yes, children can experience Brain Fog. Any and all of the conditions discussed in this book can apply to children as well as adults and must be considered before labeling a child as having Attention Deficit/Hyperactivity Disorder. It has been my experience that 80-90% of children are mislabeled as Attention Deficit Disorder (ADD) or Attention Deficit Hyperactivity Disorder (ADHD). Many people combine the two, and it is called AD/HD, where AD/HD is defined as:

- Distractibility
- Lack of focus
- Inattentiveness

Brain Fog can share the same symptoms. The difference between the two is that AD/HD is the result of a particular chemical imbalance in the brain, whereas Brain Fog is the result of other factors that make one forgetful and absent-minded.

We also need to bear in mind that AD/HD is not limited to childhood. People don't outgrow true AD/HD, rather they adapt and learn coping skills. Whether or not medicating a child will stunt his or her ability to develop coping skills is a matter for discussion elsewhere. For now, it suffices to say that we must be careful in how we diagnose our children, because a missed diagnosis of AD/HD when the child is really experiencing Brain Fog can have far reaching consequences. This book will empower you to explore the options available.

Dopamine Deficiency

True AD/HD is a deficiency of Dopamine in the brain. Dopamine is one of the major neurotransmitters that allows for focus and clarity of thought. Children who truly lack Dopamine may function better on low doses of medications such as Adderall, Ritalin, and Dexedrine. Many adults, on the other hand, have learned to self-medicate to avoid the symptoms of AD/HD. Both caffeine and nicotine metabolize into Dopamine in the brain. Smokers and heavy coffee drinkers frequently keep treating their brains to increase levels of Dopamine so that they improve their ability to function and focus.

Dopamine Deficiency Is Rare

It has been my experience that 80 to 90 percent of children diagnosed with AD/HD do not have true AD/HD. Instead, they have a dysfunction of structure, hormones, diet, or their emotional environment is disrupted. They may have nutritional deficiencies, food allergies, mercury toxicity, and basically the same problems that adults have when they complain of brain fog.

The Importance Of Making The Right Diagnosis

I have found, in over 22 years of practice, that making the right diagnosis is the principle factor in treating vague conditions such as Brain Fog and AD/HD. Many physicians just keep increasing medication until it overwhelms the brain. These high doses of stimulants override the deficiencies or imbalances that are causing the AD/HD symptoms.

What I have set out to do in this book is to make you aware of the many different factors that could be affecting your brain and hence your ability to think clearly. We will go from the simple and obvious, such as lack of sleep or lack of proper hydration, to more involved and complex issues such as hormones and toxin removal. We will look at the kind of nutritional support your brain needs and the things you can do to start the repair process so that you can best express the vitality that is really you. Brain Fog will show you how to protect, preserve and regain brain function so that you can live your life to the fullest.

CHAPTER 2

Structure and Brain Function

Susan was a 32-year-old, bright, cheerful, energetic homemaker and mother of three. When her vehicle rear-ended another vehicle at high speed, her head hit the windshield. She did not lose consciousness but she was dazed. She was told that she had a mild concussion and would be fine in a few weeks. Weeks turned into months, and months turned into years. She became progressively less functional, and remembering ordinary things became difficult. She would lose her way in familiar environments. Her temperament changed, and she became moody and somewhat depressed and irritable. Susan was afraid that she was developing dementia and would never be able to participate in normal activities again.

When I first saw Susan, I found her to have significant structural imbalances in both her head and neck. Using osteopathic manipulation, I was able to restore structural balance, which alleviated her condition and restored her brain to full function. Within four weeks, Susan started regaining her memory and ability to learn new things. Her mood changed, and she was no longer cranky. Within six weeks her husband was thankful to have rediscovered the woman he had married 10 years earlier, and her children were glad to have their happy mommy back.

One of the most fascinating areas of study is called *somato-viscero* reflexes. "Somato" refers to the body structure; i.e., the muscles and bones. "Viscero" refers to the organs within. A somato-viscero reflex refers to how your body's structure affects the organs within. This is a major principle of osteopathic medicine and holds true for a large variety of diseases and illnesses. Since the body's structure is a custom-designed encasement of the organs within, it stands to reason that alteration of the structure will affect the organs contained within that structure. Whether it is your car or your body, nothing works well if it is out of alignment or not fully mobile. For example, you cannot breathe deeply if there is a muscle spasm of the ribs, or walk well with arthritic knees. This also holds true for your brain. The musculoskeletal system can have a profound effect on the ability of your brain to function.

Before we can begin to discuss how the structure of the body affects brain function, we need to discuss a little bit of the anatomy of the head from the inside out. The brain is encased in a number of layers. The first layer of tissue to surround the brain is called the meninges. (Ever heard of meningitis? That is when the meninges are infected or inflamed.) Between the layers of the meninges is a fluid called the cerebral spinal fluid (CSF). The CSF serves to cushion, protect, and nourish the brain. This fluid is secreted from certain areas of the brain and can be found all of the way down the spinal cord. The outermost layer of the meninges is called the dura mater (dura for short). The dura is covered by the skull, which is also called the cranium. The dura's primary attachment to the cranium is where it exits the skull in the area called the foramen magnum. It then attaches to the second and third vertebrae of the neck, and finally to the second section of the sacrum, terminating in a thin little cord that extends into the coccyx (the tip of the "tailbone"). This is important to understand because it explains how a structural problem in the lower back can create a pulling effect on the dura that can reflect all the way up to the neck and into the brain resulting in headaches, neck aches, and even brain fog.

Most people think the skull is one bone, like a hard helmet. Believe it or not, the skull is not solid. It is designed for movement. There are 22 bones of the skull called the cranial bones. The cranial bones are separate, distinct bones, and they are not fused. The junctions of the cranial bones are called sutures and they are designed to move ever so slightly to accommodate the brain which is an organ that pulsates. The brain expands and contracts in a pulsating manner, curling and uncurling 8 to 12 times a minute. This expansion and contraction of the brain results in a subtle expansion and contraction of the cranium by exerting a hydraulic-like pressure via the CSF.

The ability of the cranial bones to respond to the pulsations of the brain can be impaired by a trauma such as a direct blow to the head, an imbalance in the teeth causing tempero-mandibular joint dysfunction (TMJ), muscle spasms in the neck or elsewhere in the body that pull on the fascia surrounding the skull, poorly prescribed lenses in reading glasses, and even hair pulled too tightly in a pony tail. Whatever the cause, the effect is the same. The brain will not function optimally if the cranial bones do not move freely. Fortunately, there are osteopathic techniques to enhance mobility of the cranial bones and balance structure and function. These techniques have been shown to have profound effects on mood, memory, and motivation.

Distorted cranial mobility and the consequent inhibition of the movement of the brain within have far reaching effects. Especially in children who frequently fall and hit their heads, impaired movement of the skull bones can result in the development of ear infections, sinus infections, and Attention Deficit/Hyperactivity Disorder (AD/HD). Other effects can include sluggishness, loss of enthusiasm, and mental confusion. I have often seen chronic ear infections in children clear up after 1 or 2 treatments using gentle osteopathic manipulative cranial techniques.

One of my memorable experiences was that of treating Jonathan. Jonathan was 8 years old and always getting into trouble. He was very bright but rowdy, disruptive in school, and having difficulty with his schoolwork. He was argumentative and combative. To make matters worse, he came from a broken home. His mother kicked his father out of the house 2 years earlier because of his drunken episodes. Everybody thought that Jonathan's behavior was a direct result of emotional distress. Jonathan and his mother went for counseling, but nothing changed. What everyone overlooked was that he was delivered with forceps, suffered from frequent ear infections as a toddler, and at about the age of 7 had fallen down the stairs striking his head. Two weeks after the fall, his misbehavior began. Treating him with gentle cranial osteopathy he began to sleep better, his sinus infections cleared, and he was able to pay attention in school. This remarkable response occurred in just 3 treatments.

Cranial function and its effects on the mind and body began with William Garner Sutherland when he was a senior medical student in the American School of Osteopathy in 1899. Through his intensive study of anatomy and physiology, he became aware of and fascinated by the motility of the bones of the skull. During the next 55 years of his medical career, he expanded upon this principle, researching, testing, demonstrating, and proving that the movement of the brain and the cranial bones has profound effects not only on the function of the brain but also on the function of the rest of the body.

Dr. Sutherland demonstrated how the cranial bones and their attachments to the fascia acted like the strings of a marionette, exerting profound influence on a variety, if not all, functions of the body. There are tens of thousands of stories of people who have experienced remarkable cures of a variety of ills after treatment with cranial manipulation. For example, if the symptoms of AD/HD, including poor focus and irritability, are due to a dysfunction of the cranial bones, once cranial movement is restored, the symptoms resolve within a few days.

Case Study: Jeremy

By the time Jeremy was five years old, he was diagnosed with ADHD. He could not sit still and learn the alphabet. He was always running about. He could be very moody and was short tempered and he was prone to outbursts of rage. Ritalin had been suggested when he started kindergarten, but his mother was hesitant to use the drug and instead brought Jeremy in for treatment. Jeremy's mother reported that her labor and delivery of Jeremy were very difficult, and eventually he had to be delivered with the use of forceps. Although at birth he seemed to be a normal child, within a few months he was cranky, colicky, and spitting up excessively. When I examined Jeremy, his head was very tight and his neck was stiff. He had a hard time sitting still and had to be distracted constantly. After only a few treatments of applying gentle cranial manipulation, he calmed down, rested better, focused more, and stopped acting out. His teachers thought he was a different child. The profound effect of a distorted cranium on Jeremy was such that had his mother not been proactive in investigating means to avoid medications, he would have been labeled, medicated, and significantly disadvantaged throughout his life.

Cranial Manipulation

Over the past 60 years, a number of societies have been founded to promulgate the cranial approach first begun by Dr. Sutherland. Premier in this area are the Cranial Academy and The Sutherland Cranial Teaching Foundation, which instruct both osteopathic (D.O.) and allopathic (M.D.) physicians as well as dentists in the cranial approach to alleviating structural dysfunctions. Their in-depth well-structured courses in cranial osteopathy embrace healing through structure/function relationships.

More recently, John Upledger, D.O., has offered courses to physical therapists, occupational therapists and massage therapists in Cranio-Sacral manipulation so that more people can benefit from this approach.

Regardless of whether you go to a D.O., M.D., D.D.S., D.C., P.T., or MST, treatment of the cranium should be done only by those who are experienced and well trained in the field. Movements of and pressure on the cranial bones to relieve the strain patterns of the sutures must be specific, gentle, and intentionally directed. In addition, treating the structure of the entire body is a necessary step toward the treatment of the cranium.

Case Studies: Miriam and Doug

Miriam, one of my daughter's friends, was an eight-year old little girl who had experienced some significant mood and personality changes. She had always been a very delightful, playful, productive little girl who seemingly overnight became whiny, irritable, and unable to focus. After I talked to her for a little while, it became evident that she was doing fine until the day she took a nap on the school bus, resting her head on the window of the bus. The bouncing of the bus caused her head to repeatedly bang against the window and gave her a head and neck ache. The following morning, she began having personality changes. When the restrictions of the movement of the cranial bones were alleviated and structure was rebalanced, her personality returned to its normal, happy, playful self.

I remember Doug like it was yesterday. He came in like a zombie, albeit friendly and handsome, he had a great deal of difficulty staying focused and remembering details. Doug was a history teacher and a wrestling coach at a local high school. He had brought his wrestling team to the championship finals several years in a row until he was in a car accident. Doug suffered a serious concussion and within one month was unable to remember the names of the kids in his class. He would get lost easily, his team was losing, he became temperamental, withdrawn, and irritable. Doug's problem in addition to the concussion (a severe blow to the brain which causes a bruise-like effect on the brain), was that he jammed up his cranial bones, which made it impossible for his brain to function optimally. Once the structure was corrected appropriately and the concussion treated, his memory returned, his mood elevated, he was able to function normally, needed less sleep, and he was able to apply his coaching skills to improve his team's performance.

Let us now take a look at the fascinating connective tissue of the body called the fascia. This connective tissue covers every organ and muscle in the entire body. It is a thin film that is strong and does not have the ability to stretch. It allows the muscles to slide against each other so they can move. It conveys the body's electrical forces, serves the immune system, transmits fluids, forms compartments of the body (e.g., the abdominal cavity, the thoracic cavity, and the brain cavity), defines groups of muscles, and forms ligaments and tendons. Basically the fascia connects and holds the body together. Just as pulling on the end of a sheet affects the entire sheet, strain of the fascia in one area of the body can affect an entirely different part of the body.

Knowing how the fascia connects throughout the body, you can now understand how brain fog can be caused by an injury to the tailbone (coccyx). The tailbone is often injured when someone falls on the ice or has a chair pulled out from under them when they go to sit down (children often think this is a harmless prank but a fall on the behind can injure the coccyx). You might not assume that your behind connects to your brain, but the dura is one of the meninges that extends all of the way from the brain down to the coccyx (that explains why a pain in the butt can give you a headache!). On a more serious note, an injury to that area creates a pull on the dura that can result in brain fog. Fortunately, there are gentle osteopathic manipulative techniques that can release the strain on the dura caused by the fall and your brain fog will clear. (You will also feel a whole lot better!) Even a sprained ankle can have a profound albeit indirect effect on brain function. This occurs because the fascia from the ankle goes from the ankle to the knee, to the outside of the thigh, to the buttocks, sacrum, and from there via the muscles and tendons of the spine to the skull.

What Is A Treatment?

Osteopathic treatment involves hands-on manipulation of muscles, fascia and bones. The treatment can be active, where the physician exerts force in a particular direction to release an imbalance, or so subtle that it is almost imperceptible; e.g., working on the cranium by applying gentle pressure or traction in specific areas. There are many different techniques and styles, such as muscle energy, high velocity low amplitude, low velocity high amplitude, myofascial, cranial, counterstrain, functional, ligamentous articular release, unwinding, visceral and soft tissues techniques. Sometimes treatments will involve exercise and other times may involve injections (but *never* with steroids). Basically, whatever allows the structure of the body to come into balance can be used in a treatment session. Treatments are modified to the patient and can be provided to the very young and very old alike.

Case Study: Mike

Mike was in a car accident and had a whiplash injury. For two years, he had constant headaches. When I saw him, he had been out of work for over a year because headaches prevented him from working. His headaches were so severe that he could not function. He became so irritable and belligerent that his wife was threatening divorce. He had been seen by a neurologist, orthopedist, chiropractor, and physical therapist all of whom had addressed his head and neck symptoms. My examination confirmed that although there were muscle spasms around the head and neck, there were muscle spasms all the way down to the sacrum and tailbone area. When his entire body was treated, within two months his headaches resolved entirely and he was back to working full time.

Case studies: Mendy and Jack

When I first saw Mendy, he was four months old. He cried constantly and threw up almost everything that he took in. His pediatrician had him seen by a neonatal gastroenterologist and he was diagnosed with gastroesophageal reflux disease (GERD). Medications to control the reflux were of little to no benefit. This four-month old little boy was stunted in his growth and very thin, and his parents were worn down from the constant crying and their inability to comfort the child. After I assessed the situation and his structure, I found some specific spasms and misalignments of his body and applied some corrective manipulative techniques. The child stopped crying, and that day began eating. After two more visits, his symptoms stopped entirely. He was no longer throwing up after every feeding, no longer crying incessantly, and was now able to sleep through the night.

Jack was 67 years old and had emphysema from smoking. He was on oxygen and still had difficulty breathing. He was fatigued and emaciated from spending so much energy just trying to breathe, that he was considering suicide. After I applied some basic osteopathic manipulative techniques to his upper back, ribs, and pelvis, his breathing began to ease, got deeper, and calmer. Within two weeks, he no longer needed oxygen, his fatigue lifted, and his outlook on life changed dramatically. Although he still had emphysema, his lungs could now work at their maximum efficiency, which meant that his movements and daily activities were no longer so severely restricted.

Scars

Another area that can affect skull mobility is scars. As a wound heals and begins to form a scar, the tissues that were once separated may now be drawn together like a knot. As the scar heals, it retracts and pulls on the fascia, creating a tug-like sensation on the body. This oftentimes results in a strain pattern, which affects parts of the body seemingly unrelated to the scar itself. The restriction of motion imposed on the body by a scar may not be noticed for many years. Usually an event occurs that activates the scar, such as a fall, strain or other injury, accentuating its effect on the structure and causing symptoms to develop.

I often explain the effect of scars by way of an example. Imagine yourself on a balance beam with a wind blowing from the side. As long as you are in balance you can cope with the wind, but once you stumble the wind doesn't allow you to regain your balance. The wind is the scar and the stumble can be any kind of trauma. This also explains why a scar can be dormant for years until suddenly you experience a traumatic event that triggers the scar resulting in a chronic problem.

Procaine injections to scars, called Neural Therapy, have been used for many decades. Neural Therapy is extremely safe, effective, and as an added benefit, seems to make the scar virtually disappear. I have used this therapy thousands of times and have found the relief of pain to be immediate. It rarely needs to be repeated more than two or three times.

A common scenario involves women with chronic head and/or neck aches that have previously had some type of surgery in their abdominal area, such as a cesarean section or hysterectomy. Treating their head or neck does not alleviate their pain because the problem is coming from the scars that formed from the surgery. You can understand this by tucking the front of your shirt into your pants too tightly, as you go to stand up you will feel a tug on the back of your neck. This is what you may be feeling from the scar pulling on the fascia causing pain in the head and neck area. By injecting those scars with small amounts of procaine (commonly known as Novocain) the tension and pain in the head and neck are relieved immediately.

Case Study: Samantha

Samantha had chronic headaches and was moody and irritable almost all of the time. It seems to have begun after she hurt herself doing gymnastics. She was treated by her chiropractor, but all she could get was temporary relief. After a few months, her chiropractor wisely referred her for a second opinion. Her examination was significant in that it showed that there was a scar from a cyst that was removed from her upper back years earlier. When the scar was treated by injection with procaine, her headaches went away instantly. Within two days, she was no longer moody and was back to her pleasant self.

Since the structure of your body has such far reaching effects on how it functions, I suggest getting an evaluation and, if need be, treatment by a competent osteopath who specializes in osteopathic manipulation, and who can alleviate any strain patterns your body may be holding on to.

Resources

Books

Several published books cover craniosacral mechanisms underlying the craniosacral system.

An Introduction to Craniosacral Therapy
By Don Cohen
Presents modern craniosacral therapy and describes how the structural configuration of the cranial bones affects the body.

Craniosacral Therapy
By John Upledger, D.O., and Jon Vredevoogd
Describes the rapidly growing field of therapy involving the cranial bones, meningeal membranes, cerebrospinal fluids, and whole-body connective tissues.

Dr. Fulford's Touch of Life
By Robert C. Fulford, D.O.
A fascinating insight into the philosophy and approaches utilized by one of the great healers of our time.

Additional Resource

The Cranial Academy
A resource where you can find physicians who practice osteopathy in the cranial field as well as books for the lay public and the professional. 8202 Clear Vista Parkway, #9-D Indianapolis, Indiana. 46256
(317) 584-0411
Email: cranacad@aol.com

CHAPTER 3

Stress and Fatigue

Stress and fatigue are by far the most common causes of brain fog. According to Stedman's Medical Dictionary, stress is defined as "the reactions of the animal body to forces of a deleterious nature, infections, and various abnormal states that tend to disturb its normal physiologic equilibrium." Stress is what you experience when there is an imbalance between expectations and reality. It is a term that denotes an unexpected change in or increased level of activity that exceeds an individual's capabilities.

Inadequate rest and excessive stress have very deleterious effects on brain function and can result in chronic brain dysfunction with memory loss, mood changes, irritability, and the hastening of the aging process. Either stress or fatigue will cause brain fog, or they can be the underlying causes of diseases that also result in brain fog, due to their effect on:

- Immune function
- Thyroid function
- Adrenal function
- Neurosteroids
- Behavior
- The repair process of sleep

Chronic Stress

Nearly two decades ago, a *Time Magazine* cover article called stress "the leading health problem in the United States." Repeated exposure to stress, uncertainty, lack of control, overactivity, and inadequate sleep can result in a metabolic change of the brain. Chronic stress causes prolonged activation of the body's stress response system. In this state, the brain's coping mechanism, "taxed to the max," becomes hypersensitive and will react to even a minimal amount of stress.

Physiologic Responses

Rather than concentrate on the recognition and diagnosis of individual diseases, early pioneers in stress medicine began to look at the difference between "wellness" and "illness." They researched the role of stress in the development of all types of illness.

Walter B. Cannon

A physiologist at Harvard named Walter B. Cannon was the first to describe the physiologic response to stress in the early part of the 20th century, calling it the "fight or flight response." He described an inborn response of quick energy bursts that prepare the body to fight or flee from perceived attack, harm, or threat.

Hans Selye

Hans Selye pioneered stress research in the 1930s and found that any problem, imagined or real, can cause the cerebral cortex (the thinking component of the brain) to send a stress signal to the hypothalamus (a switch for the stress response, located in the midbrain). The hypothalamus then responds by stimulating the Sympathetic Nervous System (SNS), thus causing secretion of adrenaline-type hormones that result in:

- Changes in heart rate, blood volume, and blood pressure
- Perspiration
- Cold extremities resulting from the shunting of blood toward the large muscles that help the human body fight or flee
- Pupils dilating to sharpen vision
- Acuteness in hearing

As soon as the human body decides that a situation is no longer dangerous, the brain stops sending signals to the nervous system. If the message to turn off the fight or flight response does not occur, and if the biochemical and hormonal changes that can happen during the fight or flight response continue, chronic stress can result.

Emotions and Stress

In today's society, the vast majority of individuals are under constant stress. Several international studies link chronic stress to a lack of control, or lack of acceptance of our lack of control, in daily life and more importantly over one's destiny. These studies also concluded that smoking, alcohol intake, and an unhealthy diet account for only 25% to 35% of the reasons we become ill. The rest is due to stress.

Japanese Migrant Study

Len Syme, Professor Emeritus of Epidemiology at the University of California in Berkeley, studied the influence of social support on illness and found that a lack of social support correlated with higher rates of disease. He studied Japanese migrants who moved from Japan to Hawaii to California and found a five-fold increase in illness among the migrants. Those who had adopted western ways had higher rates of disease, whereas those who retained traditional Japanese ways had rates as low as in Japan. Those with low rates of disease lived in a Japanese neighborhood, had Japanese friends, belonged to Japanese organizations, and sought the help of Japanese professionals when they needed a doctor, dentist, or lawyer.

Alameda County Study

Lisa Berkman, a professor at Harvard, also worked on a study that looked at the concept of social support and its influence on health. Berkman looked at a random sample of 7,000 residents in California and followed them over a nine-year period. Members of the sample had been studied extensively in 1965, and data was available on many aspects of their lives, including health and behavior.

In 1965, social support networks were measured with questions such as: are you married, how many close friends do you have, how often are you in contact with your friends, and do you attend a church or synagogue? Lisa found that illness from all causes appeared to be related to this simple index of a social support network. Subjects with few ties to other people had mortality rates two to five times higher in younger age groups than those with more social ties. A recent follow up of this group showed that the relationship between social support and health continues to hold.

The Volvo Study

Boredom in daily routine and time demands at work are the result of low personal control in the workplace. Both have been shown to cause stress. In a well-known study that took place in Sweden in a Volvo car plant, researchers observed that workers who produced cars on the production line experienced a lot of dissatisfaction with their job. The job consisted of having to complete repetitive tasks under the pressure of a deadline. The result was frequent absenteeism, elevated blood pressure, and job dissatisfaction.

When Volvo reorganized the work schedule into teams with flexible work roles and the ability to swap jobs, job satisfaction increased, blood pressure decreased, and the workers reported a greater sense of well-being.

Hormones and Stress

There are two basic hormonal culprits in the stress response:
* Adrenaline-type hormones
* Steroid-type hormones

Adrenaline-Type Hormones

Adrenaline-type hormones such as epinephrine, norepinephrine, and dopamine produce a state of heightened awareness. But over time and repeated exposure, they can produce cognitive dysfunction. Stress from aging also results in memory decline due to the increased level of epinephrine in the brain.

The hippocampus, which is the part of the brain that regulates our response to fear and stress, as well as learning and memory, is also the part that is most susceptible to damage by stress. The more it is damaged, the less one is able to handle stress. A vicious cycle is set up. The more stress there is, the more damage occurs and the less one is able to handle the stress, which results in more damage. Studies of children have found that these impairments can lead to problems with learning and academic achievement. New research has shown that the hippocampus has the capacity to regenerate nerve cells as part of its normal functioning, but stress may impair this function by slowing down the regeneration of neurons.

Steroid-Type Hormones

Stress also causes the secretion of glucocorticoids (steroids) that at first enhance the function of the hippocampus. However, with prolonged and repeated stress, glucocorticoids injure the hippocampus, causing further memory impairment. Researchers have found that different kinds of stress result in oxidative damage to different parts of the brain and to varying degrees. Oxidative damage from stress and aging destroy brain tissue, resulting in loss of function.

Signs of Stress

Stress is not necessarily bad. It can also be caused by good news that results in much rejoicing and celebration. Stress has its benefits. Stress can stimulate us to change and grow. Stress can also keep us from getting bored. Too much stress, however, is a bad thing regardless of the cause. When one becomes overstressed it can affect the mind, body, and spirit.

Stress Questionnaire

The following questionnaire will help you assess your level of stress:

Directions
Fill in a value after each question using the following as a guide:

    0   = No
    1   = Rarely
    2   = Sometimes
    3   = Always

Question	0	1	2	3
1. Are you moody or depressed?				
2. Do you have problems concentrating?				
3. Do you have aches or pains?				
4. Do you have problems sleeping?				
5. Do you drink alcohol or smoke to calm your nerves?				
6. Do you feel on edge or nervous?				
7. Do you feel rushed?				
8. Do you feel worn out?				
9. Do you lose your patience easily?				
10. Do you feel scattered or unorganized?				

Calculating Your Score

Add the numeric value of your ten responses. If your total score falls below five, you have a low amount of stress or are coping with stress well. If your score falls between 6 and 15, you may have a high amount of stress, and if your score is greater than 15, you are very likely to have severe stress which requires immediate attention.

Cranial Manipulation

Sometimes the changes in the brain caused by stress are such that medical intervention is necessary. The list of intervention possibilities is quite long, ranging from western medical approaches, acupuncture, and homeopathy, to neurochemical balancing.

Below, I will discuss four basic treatments that I have found to be helpful in the treatment of stress.

Acupuncture

The ancient Chinese treatment of placing needles in distinct areas of the body is very effective in relieving stress. However, it requires a skilled acupuncturist, a willing patient, effort, and time. There are various schools of acupuncture and a variety of techniques and approaches. There might be momentary discomfort on insertion of the needle, but once the needles are placed the patient should feel no pain.

Homeopathy

Homeopathy is the science of treating ailments with the diluted concentrations of substances that cause those ailments. For example, coffee can make you feel alert, agitated or irritable. Homeopathic coffee (caffea cruda) calms the mind, eases anxiety, and helps you fall asleep. By homeopathically diluting substances, remedies are created to balance the body and alleviate ills without the toxic effects of medications. It is very effective and must be specific to the patient. One can utilize various remedies for first aid, but for more complicated or chronic conditions, a skilled homeopath should be consulted.

Western Medical Approaches

The Western medical approach alleviates symptoms by using manufactured medicines whose effectiveness has been proven by studies on large groups of people. Although the Western medical approach can be very therapeutic, it is rarely curative and tends to create a dependency on medications.

The most common "stress pill" of all time is diazepam i.e., Valium®. This drug is designed to stimulate the GABA receptor in the brain, causing a sensation of relaxation and calm. One should use only a low dose of the medication (5 mg.or less) and only once a day. Higher and frequent doses of this medication usually mean that this is not the appropriate treatment for the condition, and dependency on the drug can be created. For a more natural approach, you can try 500-1000 mg. of Inositol 1-3 times a day to stimulate the GABA receptor in the brain.

Neurochemical Balancing

In the early 1900s, a physician in Bucharest, Romania, Ana Aslan, M.D., discovered that Procaine (the chemical name for Novocain®) was effective as an anti-aging agent as well as an antidepressant and neurochemical balancer. Volumes have been written on this subject, and studies verify its effectiveness. In brief, the Procaine formula called Gerovital H3 (GH-3) is metabolized into two essential chemicals in the body: PABA and DMAE. These two naturally occurring chemicals combine to quell the autonomic nervous system, improving one's stress response, calming nerves, and lowering anxiety from a "high-pitched scream" down to a "hum." Originally and ideally, GH3 is given by injection once every other day for a month. Then, you alternate—one month off, one month on. A pill form has been developed which is more convenient but less effective. This treatment needs to be administered under the guidance of a physician familiar with GH-3.

Free Radicals and Stress

Stress affects the body not only by altering neurochemical and hormonal balances, but also through production of free radicals. Free radicals are normal byproducts of metabolism and tend to be very destructive by nature. Free radicals can destroy tissues and alter function because of the way they affect cells and structures within the cells. One of the reasons that stress affects a person as he or she ages is due to the production of free radicals. By taking free radical scavengers and antioxidants, you can mitigate the effect of stress as well as slow down the aging progress.

To ease the effect that free radicals have on the body, I recommend taking the following with food:

- Vitamin C—500 to 1000 mg. twice a day
- Vitamin E—400 to 600 units once a day
- A good B-Complex multi-vitamin
- Alpha Lipoic Acid—100 to 200 mg. a day
- Selenium—100 to 200 mcgs. a day
- Zinc—30 mg. a day
- Copper—3 mg. a day

Self-Help: Sleep

Sleep is absolutely necessary to rejuvenate one's self, be it physically, mentally, or emotionally. Sleep deprivation and excessive stress have very deleterious effects on brain function and can result in chronic brain dysfunction with memory loss, mood changes, irritability, and hastening of the aging process.

Stages of Sleep

When one sleeps, one goes through various stages. The two most important stages are known as non-REM and REM sleep. REM stands for *rapid eye movement*.

Non-REM sleep

Delta sleep, or deep sleep, is called non-REM sleep or NREM sleep. This type of sleep is associated with physical recovery and restoration. Those who are deprived of delta sleep feel a malaise. During NREM sleep, the body temperature decreases, as does cerebral blood flow. There are also declines in the metabolic rates for glucose uptake, as well as declines in cortisol levels and oxygen consumption. During NREM sleep, growth hormone and pro-lactin levels increase.

REM sleep

REM sleep is characterized by dreaming and rapid eye movement beneath closed eyelids. REM sleep occurs approximately every 90 minutes and lasts from 5 to 30 minutes. During REM sleep, body temperature, glucose and oxygen consumption rise to almost waking levels. This stage is also characterized by a decrease in the Thyroid Stimulating Hormone (TSH), an increase in cortisol levels and testosterone (particularly in males), and an increase in Melatonin.

Sleep has restorative properties due to a change in metabolism and hormones. Sleep helps to maintain the synaptic neuronal network's integrity. In other words, it helps the brain to function better. During REM sleep, memory reinforcement and consolidation occur, thereby enhancing recall for the next day.

In adults, food consumed at night will alter the hormone levels of the brain. Growth hormone and testosterone are decreased while insulin and cortisol increase, altering a person's sleep cycles and making their sleep less restful and restorative. Optimally, one should not eat food of any sort after 8:00 p.m. The earlier before bedtime one stops eating, the better. However, babies and young children may need a bedtime snack in order to sleep through the night.

The Effects of Sleep Deprivation

In modern industrial societies, an average night's sleep has decreased from about nine hours in 1910 to 7.5 hours in 1975, and this trend continues. Researchers from the University of Chicago Medical Center have found that sleep loss can impair basic metabolic functions such as processing and storing carbohydrates and hormone secretion. The study, which focused on chronic, partial sleep loss, showed that cutting back from eight hours to four hours of sleep produced changes in glucose tolerance and endocrine function. In less than one week, the changes that were observed were similar to the effects of advanced age or the early stages of diabetes.

Effects of sleep deprivation include:

Learning
Studies by the United States Army on the effects of sleep deprivation showed a diminished ability to learn new things. Detailed tasks became more difficult to perform. People got irritable, impatient, and intolerant when fatigued.

Obesity
Hormonal changes in glucose tolerance due to lack of sleep can lead to weight gain. Overweight people do not sleep well. When one is overweight, there is an increased tendency for:

* Snoring
* Sleep apnea
* Nocturia (urinating at night)
* Diabetes
* Poor circulation
* Hormonal imbalances

Of these conditions, sleep apnea is the most dangerous. People who suffer from sleep apnea stop breathing dozens of times during the night and may not breathe for as much as three fourths of the time they are asleep. People with sleep apnea are tired regardless of how much they sleep. They never feel energized and doze off easily during the daytime, especially when doing an uninteresting activity.

A classic example of a sleep apnea sufferer is a middle-aged man who is 60 pounds overweight, snores heavily, has to force himself to get through the day, and is never refreshed or energetic. He likes to nosh, and the minute he gets the least bit bored he falls asleep—whether reading the paper, driving, or sitting in a meeting.

Pain
When one is hurting or ill, there is a strain on the immune system and more sleep is required. Furthermore, a tired person is more likely to feel pain or to become injured or ill because of a weakened immune system. Extra rest is required for recovery from illness or injury.

Physical Activity
High levels of physical activity demand more sleep. If workers or athletes do not get the sleep they need, not only do they lose strength but they are more prone to injuries and their performance suffers.

Important Note: Fatigue is one of the two most common causes of injuries both in sports and on the job. The other most common cause is dehydration from inadequate water intake.

Depression
Depression is not about being sad but about having depressed brain function. People who have been pushed to their limit and have exhausted the brain's capability to rejuvenate become depressed. Depression is the result of a chemical change in the brain that not only dulls function but also dulls one's sense of pleasure. Adequate rest during times of stress is crucial to prevent depression. However, once one is depressed rest is not the answer. Appropriate treatment of depression to restore chemical imbalances is usually necessary and may require medications. Exercise, which releases endorphins, has been shown to be effective in helping someone who is depressed.

How Much Sleep Does One Need?

The average adult should not need more than eight hours of sleep unless there is a significant alteration in energy output, such as athletic competition, increased stress, severe injury, or illness. Some people need only five to six hours of sleep, especially if they are sedentary. The key principle to bear in mind is that after a good night's rest one should feel refreshed and energized, and should not need caffeine to feel wide awake and functional.

Self-Help: Exercise

Exercise is one of the best remedies for stress. Since stress causes a fight-or-flight response in the body, exercise provides a means to channel excess energy from the stress response into a physical activity. Vigorous exercise produces substances called endorphins that induce feelings of well-being and relaxation. Endorphins have a chemical structure similar to that of morphine. You may find that exercise has a relaxation effect so that at bedtime you will fall asleep faster.

Walking is a Simple Way to Unwind

Many people consider walking to be the perfect exercise. It is an exercise that does not require athletic ability, it is very low risk, and it puts minimal stress on the body. Brisk walking:

- Releases endorphins
- Lowers blood pressure
- Burns off calories
- Improves circulation
- Lowers blood sugar in diabetics
- Improves memory
- Prevents and reverses osteoporosis
- Is inexpensive
- Can be shared with a friend
- Produces a sense of well-being

Consider the following tips:

Find Someone to Walk With
Sharing a nice long walk with a friend is a fun way to socialize.

Join a Walking or Hiking Club
If you have trouble finding someone to share a walk, consider joining a walking or hiking club.

Choose a Comfortable Pair of Shoes
Walking requires comfortable, supportive walking shoes. Try to find a waterproof pair so you won't be put off by walking in the rain, and look for

cushioning if you plan to walk on concrete sidewalks. If you walk on natural paths, you may prefer a pair of lightweight hiking shoes.

Dress for the Weather
Layered clothing is practical in hot weather or cold. Choose fabrics that breathe.

Plan Your Route
Your first concern when you plan your route should be safety. Plan a familiar route through major cross streets and intersections that can help you get your bearings if you make a wrong turn. Look for points of interest such as parks, historic areas, or shopping districts. Many people like to combine errands with their walks.

Walk Vigorously
Walking at any pace is good, but walking vigorously is best. Not only does it help burn off more calories and increase your muscle tone faster, but it helps produce endorphins and has generally been found to be more effective in stress reduction.

Self Help: Yoga

Hatha yoga is the most widely practiced form of yoga in America and many find it to be a pleasant antidote to stress. It is a branch of yoga that uses bodily postures *(asanas)*, breathing techniques *(pranayama)*, and meditation *(dyana)* to create a sound, healthy body and a clear, peaceful mind. There are nearly 200 Hatha yoga postures, with hundreds of variations, which work to make the spine supple and to promote circulation in all the organs, glands, and tissues. Hatha yoga postures also stretch and align the body, promoting balance and flexibility.

Postures and Breathing
Yoga asanas consist of three basic movements:

- Backward bends
- Forward bends
- Twisting movements

Postures are always balanced with a forward bend following a back bend and a right movement following a left movement. Diaphragmatic breathing, with breath beginning at the bottom of the lungs, is important during the pose. The stomach moves outward with inhalation and relaxes inward during exhalation. Breath is accomplished through the nose at all times during hatha asanas, with inhales during backward bends and exhales during forward bends.

The combination of specific movements, muscle contraction, controlled breathing, and focused attention provides a sense of relaxation and calm. This calming effect combined with muscle toning and increased flexibility has a significant effect on the ability to manage stress throughout the day.

Self Help: Vacations

In a study published in the April 2000 edition of the *Journal of Occupational Medicine,* an Austrian research team found that employees of a manufacturing company reported fewer physical complaints for five weeks after their return from vacation.

Vacations and periods of relaxation are not luxuries—they are necessities. This was driven home to me years ago while I was still in school. After some particularly trying semesters, I found that it was difficult to absorb information when I read, and even remembering phone numbers was difficult. I was not sleeping well and I was irritable. When I took a vacation, all of these symptoms seemed to melt away. Within seven days, my stress began to disappear. I began breathing deeper, my speech became clearer, and my mental processes sharpened. I experienced a renewed interest in reading and learning. After ten days, I felt like a new man. Once I was back from vacation, people commented that I looked more relaxed and younger.

I felt stronger, more alert, and my mood was up. I felt full of pizzazz. One needs a period of respite from stresses and strains to regenerate the brain, to renew and refresh. Such reinvigoration helps one return to life with joy and vitality.

Tips for a Stress-Free Vacation

If you are seeking a relaxing holiday, the following tips can help make your vacation as stress-free as possible.

Choose a Restful Destination

If low stress is your goal, choose a restful travel destination over a tour vacation. Moving from one destination to the next every couple of days is not restful.

Limit Your Sun Exposure

A bad case of sunburn can create stress and ruin a well-deserved vacation. Too much sun exposure can tax the nervous and endocrine systems and leave you feeling tired and washed out. If you are going to the beach, use a beach umbrella. Protect your eyes with sunglasses that offer UV protection. Drink plenty of fluids so you don't get dehydrated.

"HOT TIP:"—You can tell when you are drinking enough fluids because your urine is clear.

Focus on the Moment

Minimize your expectations while you are away. Focus on the moment and have fun.

Plan Within Your Budget

Financial issues may be a source of stress for people on holidays. If you're on a budget, select destinations that will not stretch your pocketbook.

Allow Plenty of Traveling Time

Give yourself plenty of traveling time for the trip. Plan your itinerary so you don't have to rush to catch airplanes or trains. Allow time to come home, unpack, readjust, take in the mail, and get the phone messages so that life can begin at a normal easy pace. Many people schedule time at work after a vacation to catch up on their mail, email and phone messages.

Don't Over-Schedule

Don't overload your schedule so that you are overtired. Allow plenty of time for spontaneous activity.

Self-Help: Amino Acid

Although the anxiety response is vital for our survival, it can inflict physical degeneration on our bodies. Amino acids can relieve anxiety and strengthen the nervous system. Amino acids are building blocks the body uses to make protein.

The body continuously breaks down proteins into amino acids, which it then recombines to form whatever proteins it needs to maintain itself. Amino acids supply the raw materials for maintaining DNA, muscle tissue, enzymes, connective tissue, hormones, and neurotransmitters.

Amino Acid	Description
Histidine	Histidine is a precursor of histamine that has a stimulating effect on the nervous system, changing brain waves from beta-dominated to alpha. Histidine works well with Niacin and B6 and an equal quantity of C (ascorbic acid). Histidine should not be given to manic depressives or people with high levels of histamine.
Tryptophan	Tryptophan is a precursor to the sleep-inducing neurotransmitter serotonin and works to relieve anxiety. It is also a precursor to vitamin B3 (niacin). A lack of B3 causes nervousness, irritability, and anxiety. In the 1950s, psychiatrist Dr. Abram Hoffer and his colleagues researched the biochemistry of schizophrenia and proposed a restorative treatment using vitamins B3 and C. He used 3,000 mg of vitamin B3 with 3,000 mg. of vitamin C, and many recovered.

Glycine	Glycine has a calming effect on the mind. It is used by the body to make glutathione, which is involved in the body's detoxification pathways and the immune system. Glycine plays an important role in wound healing and the immune system. It has a sweet taste and is used as a food additive.
Taurine	Taurine is vital to the proper utilization of sodium, magnesium, potassium, and calcium, and has a protective effect upon the human brain. The amino acid taurine is used to treat anxiety, hyperactivity, poor brain function, hypoglycemia, epilepsy, hypertension, and seizures.
5-HTP (Hydroxy Tryptophan)	5-HTP is a precursor to serotonin particularly in the brain. It is very useful for people who have a difficult time staying asleep through the night. It has also been shown to reduce anxiety that can lead to overeating. Compulsive overeaters may often benefit from taking 5-HTP even in small doses of 25 mg. to 50 mg. Occasionally, a higher dose of 150 mg. is needed twice a day. A nighttime dose that helps people stay asleep through the night is 50 to 200 mg. 5-HTP has been found to be safe up to 300 mg.

Self-Help: Herbs

There are several herbs that are known to reduce stress and anxiety. Herbs are nature's pharmacy. They are commercially available as bulk teas, bagged teas, herbal capsules, and liquid tinctures.

Herb	Description
Chamomile	A member of the daisy family, tea made from this herb has a mild sedative effect.
Ginseng	Ginseng root contains active ingredients called ginsenosides. Of these, the Rb and Rg ginsenosides are the most significant. Rb-1 has the yin quality of a calming effect on the body, helping it manage stress, while Rg-1 has a yang effect of stimulating the body, thus giving it energy. Taken together, ginseng's ginsendosides restore memory and raise tolerance to physical and psychological stress. American Ginseng is an adaptogen that can serve to calm the nerves and Siberian or Korean Ginseng helps the body endure high levels of activity and enhance energy.
Kava Kava	Kava Kava has become the most popular herb for relieving anxiety. In 1990, Germany's Commision E (equivalent to the FDA) approved Kava Kava for treating anxiety and stress. Long-term use may cause allergic reactions, visual disturbances, and liver toxicity. Use of this herb should not exceed three consecutive months.
Licorice Root	Licorice root is an adaptogen that works in a non-specific way to normalize the actions of the organs and protect them from chronic stress. Licorice root strengthens the nervous, immune, and endocrine systems. Because of licorice root's tendency to elevate the blood pressure in people with hypertension, one must be cautious when using this herb. This is particularly true in people who retain fluids or have high blood pressure. Licorice root is most helpful in people with low blood pressure.

St. John's Wort	St. John's Wort has been found to work as well as prescription antidepressants for treating mild to moderate depression. Side effects include possible weight gain and sensitivity to light. The herb is thought to increase serotonin levels in the brain and should not be taken with drugs that affect serotonin levels, including SSRIs (Selective Seratonin Reuptake Inhibitors such as Prozac, Paxil, Zoloft, etc.), SAMe or Monamine Oxidase Inhibitors (MAOIs).
Valerian	Animal studies have shown that valerian root is an effective stress reducer and sedative. Very high doses can cause headaches, muscle spasms and insomnia. Long-term use can also cause liver damage.
Hops	Hops are used in the brewing industry to give beer flavor. The herb is a distant relative of marijuana and is considered a remedy for anxiety and insomnia. Some manufacturers combine hops with valerian root, as one study showed the two herbs have synergistic interaction.
Passionflower	Passionflower has been shown to reduce anxiety, insomnia, and high blood pressure. One study found the herb to be as effective as Valium but without the sedative side effects.

Self Help: Aromatherapy

Aromatherapy is a holistic treatment using botanical oils made from plants. Oils can be used to alleviate tension and fatigue, relieve pain, invigorate the body, or for skin care. When inhaled, essential oils work on the brain and nervous system through stimulation of the olfactory nerves.

The Greeks, Romans, and ancient Egyptians all used aromatherapy oils. In the 1930s, French chemist Rene Maurice Gattefosse coined the term aromatherapy when he used lavender oil to heal his burned hand. He started investigating the effect of other essential oils for healing and other psychotherapeutic benefits.

Essential Oil	Description
Lavender	Relaxes and relieves stress
Rosemary	Sharpens the mind
Geranium	Reduces stress
Chamomile	Reduces stress
Clary sage	Relaxes and relieves stress
Sandalwood	Good for insomnia and depression
Juniper berry	Good for reducing anxiety and anger
Sweet marjoram	Reduces anxiety

How to Use Essential Oils

Although essential oils are plant essences, they must be used carefully. Oils should never be swallowed, and care should be taken not to touch one's eyes if there is any oil residue on one's fingers. All oils will eventually deteriorate. It is best to store oils in a cool, dark place. If you store oils in the refrigerator, keep them separated from food in an airtight container.

Citrus oils have a shelf life of six months and other oils will keep for one year. Oils may be used actively or passively. Active methods include use in the bath, in massage, and in hot and cold compresses. Oils may also be used passively by spreading the fragrance into a room. This is accomplished with light bulb rings, aromatherapy candles, ceramic vaporizers, and pump sprays that mix the oil with water.

Oils that are used directly on the skin should be diluted with a carrier oil. Examples of carrier oils include sweet almond or jojoba. To dilute an essential oil, you will need a clean, dark glass bottle. Measure 4 teaspoons of a carrier oil and add up to 10 drops of an essential oil for direct application to the skin *(See: Resources, Product, Essential Oil)*.

Self-Help: Music

Ancient cultures knew that music and sound affect the body, mind, and spirit. Recent studies of psychological responses to music in the relaxation process have been overwhelmingly positive. Music can play an important role in the treatment of persons suffering from stress-related disorders. It has been demonstrated that music can dramatically influence physiological and psychological processes.

Dr. Alfred Tomatis

Dr. Alfred Tomatis, a French ear, nose and throat specialist, uses music, chants and various tones to treat people with autism and obsessive disorders. He discovered the power of chant after visiting a Benedictine monastery in France. The monks had stopped chanting because the new abbot believed that the Gregorian chant served no useful purpose. When the chanting stopped, the monks became more and more tired. Doctors tried to restore their energy with diet and sleep but to no avail. Tomatis reintroduced the chanting and within nine months, almost all the monks had their energy back. They were able to resume normal activities that included prayer, a few hours of sleep, and an arduous work schedule.

Dr. Masaru Emoto

Japanese researcher and author of *The Message From Water,* Dr. Masaru Emoto, Ph.D. studied the differences in the crystalline structures of water molecules that react to human vibrational energy, thoughts, ideas, and music. His photographs offer proof that water reacts to environmental conditions as well as to thoughts, feelings, and sound. By freezing droplets of water and photographing them under a dark field microscope, he noticed major differences in the appearance of crystals.

This experiment was repeated many times over with the same result. When he exposed water samples to different types of music, classical music always reflected beautiful patterns, whereas heavy metal or rock and roll created distorted, formless, and smudged images, as if these types of music had destroyed the equilibrium of the molecules.

Inspired by these results, he decided to study the impact of human consciousness on water and its crystalline order. For example, he found that water molecules could be imprinted. He accomplished this by adding words to water jars with paper. Water that was imprinted with the words "love," "gratitude," and "appreciation" resulted in crystals with complex beauty whereas water that was imprinted with negative intentions became distorted and grotesque. *(To see Dr. Masaru Emoto's images, look for the Web address in this chapter under Resources, Research, Dr. Masaru Emoto.)*

Resources

Alliances and Organizations

Alliances and organizations that provide valuable up-to-date information include:

The American Institute of Stress
124 Park Avenue
Yonkers, NY 10703
(914) 963-1200 stress125@earthlink.net
www.stress.org
AIS provides information on various types of stress as well as a monthly newsletter and expert consultation on-line.

Parent's Anonymous, Inc.
675 W. Foothill Blvd, Suite 220
Claremont, CA 91711
(909) 621-6184
parentsanon@voiceofwomen.com
www.voiceofwomen.com/parents/anon.html

Maryland Chapter
(410) 243-7337 or (800) 243-7337
A self-help group for parents and children providing education and support in an effort to prevent child abuse. Many publications for new mothers and families, as well as a 24-hour stress hotline.

Prevent Child Abuse America
200 S. Michigan Avenue
17th Floor
Chicago, IL 60604-2404
(312) 663-3520
www.preventchildabuse.org

Survivors of Incest Anonymous
World Service Office
P.O. Box 190
Benson, MD 21018
(410) 893-3322
www.siawso.org

National Organization for Victim Assistance
1730 Park Road, NW
Washington, DC 20010
(202) 232-6682
(800) TRY-NOVA
www.try-nova.org

The American Yoga Association
P.O. Box 19986
Sarasota, FL 34276
(941) 927-4977
www.americanyogaassociation.org
A nonprofit organization that is a resource for both yoga students and teachers. The American Yoga Association offers a free online yoga lesson every month.

*Rich and Char Tosi
Couples Weekends
Phenomenal weekends designed for healing and growth for couples.
(810) 750-7227
couples@tosi.biz

www.tosi.biz
*The Mankind Project
Non-sectarian, weekend retreats for self-discovery. Sponsors the New Warrior Training for Men.
Drury Heffernan, Network Administrator
Phone (800) 870-4611
Fax (514) 624-2527
PO Box 230
Malone NY 12953-0230
E-Mail: drury@mkp.org
1-800-870-4611
www.mkp.org

*Woman Within International
Weekend retreats for self-discovery and healing. Sponsors Woman Within Training.
www.womanwithin.org
Woman Within International, Ltd.
P.O. Box 441494
Detroit, MI 48244
(800) 732-0890
On the East Coast contact:
www.ecsagecircle.org
Christel Libiot, East Coast Sage Circle Administrator
(301) 372-8718
or Christel1@att.net
East Coast Sage Circle also sponsors Woman Within Training.

Tierra Marketing—TMI
223 North Guadalupe
Suite #285
Santa Fe, NM 87501
(800) 736-6253
www.realgh3.com

International Anti-Aging Systems
IAS Limited
Les Autelets #B
Sark GY9 0SF
Great Britain
www.antiaging-systems.com

Book

GH3: Will It Keep You Young Longer?
By: Herbert Bailey
Published by: Cancer Book House
Herbert Baily covers GH3 developed by Dr. Ana Aslan, a Romanian physician who specialized in studies of gerontology, geriatrics and cardiology. Her GH3 formula contains procaine hydrochloride that has proven beneficial side effects to people suffering from a range of ailments.

*I recommend these very highly.

CHAPTER 4

Hypothyroidism

Many of the problems of aging, such as achiness, constipation, weight gain, brain fog, moodiness, dry skin, slow metabolism, and feeling cold are often associated with low thyroid, also known as hypothyroidism. The thyroid is a gland in the neck that produces several hormones, including Thyroxine (T4) and Triiodothyronine (T3). These two hormones are responsible for making the thyroid gland the *master gland of metabolism* because they regulate energy production in the body by controlling the rate at which cells produce and consume energy.

A hormone is a molecular "messenger" that is sent through the bloodstream to tell the cells how to function. For example, once the thyroid gland produces Thyroxine (T4) and Triiodothyronine (T3), these hormones enter the blood stream and cause the brain to think, bowels to move, heart to beat, joints to be fluid, skin to be soft, nails to be hard, energy of the body to be increased, and sleep to be restorative.

Symptoms of Hypothyroidism (Low Thyroid)

Although your doctor will need to help you determine if you have an underactive thyroid, the following list of symptoms can alert you that you may have a problem:

Fatigue

No matter how much you sleep, if you are low on thyroid, you will wake up feeling tired. However, people with low thyroid find that once they start moving, they feel better. Activity makes low thyroid patients feel more energized, and rest makes them feel more fatigued.

Brain Fog

Spaciness, confusion, forgetfulness and an inability to focus are all symptoms of brain fog that may be caused by low thyroid function.

Depression

Too little thyroid may cause depression as well as paranoia and dementia.

Cold Intolerance

Low energy production in the body may cause the body to feel cold. People with low thyroid feel cold even though everyone else feels warm.

Constipation

Because thyroid hormones enhance peristalsis or movement of the intestinal tract, low thyroid can result in constipation.

Night Blindness

Difficulty seeing at night can be caused by low thyroid.

Hearing Loss

Inadequate amounts of thyroid hormone in the body affect hearing and can lead to hearing loss.

Weight Gain or An Inability to Lose Weight

Thyroid hormones impact the production of growth hormones. Low thyroid results in low growth hormone production causing an increased amount of fat and decreased lean body mass. To make matters worse, dieting and exercise seem to have little impact on those with an underactive thyroid.

Elevated Cholesterol

People with low thyroid tend to have an increase in LDL or low-density lipoprotein (the bad cholesterol), and a decrease in the HDL or high-density lipoprotein (the good cholesterol).

Hair, Skin and Nail Problems

Dry skin and brittle nails are a common consequence of low thyroid.

Irregular Menstrual Cycles (heavy or more frequent)

Menstrual irregularities are very common with hypothyroidism.

Menopause

Hypothyroidism may become worse during menopause, and is most common in women between the ages of 40 and 60. Women in this age group should be carefully screened for hypothyroidism because symptoms of hypothyroidism and menopause are very similar.

Snoring or Sleep Apnea

Obesity caused by hypothyroidism can result in snoring and/or sleep apnea. In addition, the fatigue caused by sleep apnea and snoring stresses the body even further, making hypothyroidism worse.

Aches in Joints including Carpal Tunnel Syndrome (CTS)

Achy joints and stiff muscles are very common symptoms of hypothyroidism. People with hypothyroidism find that as long as they are in motion, they feel fine, but once they stop moving, it is hard to start again.

Causes of Hypothyroidism (Low Thyroid)

Inadequate Iodine in the Diet

T4 and T3 refer to the number of iodine atoms attached to the hormone. T4 refers to four iodine atoms and T3 refers to three iodine atoms. Too little iodine can cause hypothyroidism and is usually associated with an enlarged thyroid gland that is called a *goiter*. Interestingly, too much iodine can also shut down the thyroid gland in much the same way as too little iodine.

Exposure to Radiation

Radiation exposure to gamma rays or x-rays can cause hypothyroidism. Anyone who has had excessive dental x-rays, been treated with x-rays for acne, or for sinusitis with radium sticks (they used to do this from the 1940s through the 1960s), or CT scans of the head as a child is at risk of developing thyroid problems and even thyroid cancer. Populations that have been exposed to nuclear radiation, such as Chernobyl in the Ukraine, Tokaimura in Japan, the Nevada deserts and Hanford in south central Washington, have experienced radiation-induced hypothyroidism.

High Consumption of Soy

Soy can interfere with thyroid function because it blocks absorption of iodine by the thyroid gland. People who have hypothyroidism should avoid high intakes of soy products unless the soy has been fermented, and then only in moderation.

High Consumption of Goitrogenic Foods

The following raw vegetables contain enzymes that depress the thyroid:

- Brussel sprouts
- Rutabaga
- Turnips
- Cauliflower
- African Cassava
- Babassu (palm-tree nut found in Brazil and Africa)
- Cabbage
- Kale

Thorough cooking will destroy the goitrogenic enzymes, making these vegetables safe to eat.

Medications

Drugs that can cause hypothyroidism include:

- Lithium
- HCTZ (Hydrochlorothiazide)
- Birth control pills
- Levadopa for Parkinson's disease

- Amiodarone for heart problems
- Growth hormones for anti-aging treatments
- Diuretics

Stress

Stress is probably the most common cause of hypothyroidism. It can be any kind of prolonged stress, including emotional stress, overexertion, trauma, overtraining in athletes, inadequate sleep, dieting, and severe caloric restriction, such as in starvation or anorexia.

Pregnancy

Pregnancy is a common cause of hypothyroidism and can result in post-partum depression.

Aging

The thyroid is a gland, and like any other gland in the body it tends with age to slow down its production of hormones.

Questioning Normal Limits

People often comment, "My doctor says my thyroid tests are normal." I have found, however, that many doctors do not accurately assess a patient's thyroid function. It is surprising how many doctors will assess a patient's thyroid solely on the range of values defined by a laboratory. For example, a normal TSH value is often considered to range from 0.5 to 5.5 (as of late 2004, the new recommendation for TSH is 0.5 to 2.5). Normal limits, however, fail to define optimal levels. What can be normal for one person is abnormal for someone else. Only when one takes into account the levels of Free T3, Free T4, and TSH in conjunction with symptoms and an appropriate physical examination, can one make an accurate diagnosis and assessment of the thyroid state.

Evaluating Your TSH Level

TSH, which stands for Thyroid Stimulating Hormone, is a hormone produced by the pituitary gland in the brain that tells the thyroid gland how hard it has to work to produce the necessary thyroid hormones T4 (Thyroxine) and T3 (Triiodothyronine). Give a good horse a little nudge and he's off. If you have to beat the horse to get him to move, there is a problem with the horse. TSH works the same way. If the thyroid is healthy, a low amount of TSH is all that is needed to make it respond. Ideally, the level should be between 0.4 and 1.0. If the thyroid is not in a healthy state, and the TSH goes above 1.0 and especially if it goes above 2.0, then the brain is working too hard to make the thyroid do too little. Not only are you susceptible to fatigue, exhaustion, and other hypothyroid symptoms, but you also run the risk of osteoporosis.

There Is More to This Story

When the TSH stimulates the thyroid gland to produce thyroid hormone, the thyroid gland produces 80 percent T4 and 20 percent T3. Ninety-five percent of these hormones are immediately bound to proteins to render them inactive in order to create a "reservoir" to tap into when needed. This is a necessary safeguard against too much thyroid flooding the body.

- *Three hormones have a role in your thyroid health: TSH, T4, and T3*
- *All hormones are either bound, i.e., inactive, or unbound, i.e., active*

Now, herein lays the problem when assessing thyroid function. The inactive thyroid hormones are measurable, and can therefore give a false reading of hormone status if all that is measured is the total hormone level.

Many doctors measure only the total thyroid hormone levels, which take into account both the bound and the unbound levels together. So, if someone has a high level of bound hormone plus a low level of unbound hormone, the results may be normal but the person may be functionally hypothyroid. Again, a free hormone—in this case thyroid hormone—is the active form of the hormone. Hormones are active only when they are not bound to a protein carrier. The free form of thyroid is "looking for action." Therefore, it is imperative when assessing thyroid function to measure Free T4 and Free T3. Measuring anything else is woefully inadequate as a means of assessing thyroid function.

Questioning Your Test Results

The bottom line is this, if your doctor tells you that your thyroid is fine after evaluating only the TSH and Total Thyroid Hormone levels, you still may be functionally hypothyroid. Therefore, you may want to make sure that your doctor takes the following into account:

1. Without evaluating Free T3 and Free T4, you cannot accurately evaluate thyroid function. Remember that only the unbound form of thyroid hormone is active and can exert an effect on the cells to increase metabolism.
2. If you have the symptoms of hypothyroidism and the blood tests are "normal," the interpretation of the blood test may be wrong.
3. Normal ranges of limits are very broad, so what is normal for one person can be abnormal for someone else.

Do not be "married" to a diagnosis of hypothyroidism. There may be other causes for your symptoms; e.g., low levels of cortisol production, depression, neurochemical imbalances, menopausal or andropausal symptoms, nutritional deficiencies, immune system dysfunction, infections, or malabsorption, to name a few. You will need an astute doctor to help figure out the vast array of possibilities for your symptoms. Do not be afraid to look elsewhere.

Your T4 to T3 Ratio

The T4 to T3 ratio is very important for evaluating thyroid hormone function. It tells us how efficiently the body is converting T4 into T3—that is, converting the reservoir into the active hormone. The ratio of Free T3 to Free T4 should be between 0.3 to 0.35. About 30 to 35 percent of the Free Thyroid Hormone in the blood should be Free T3. The lower the ratio of Free T3 to Free T4, the less efficient is the conversion of T4 into T3 and the more fatigued a person feels.

Normal Ranges	TSH	Free T4	Free T3
(May vary slightly between labs)	0.4-3.0	0.9-1.4 ngs/dl	0.287-0.55 ngs/dl

Case Studies: Carol, Bob, Betty, Brenda, and Mary

Carol always woke up tired and was sluggish throughout the day. Sleep did not seem to help. She felt better when she was active and moving, but it was hard for her to get started. Blood tests showed that her TSH was 2.1, the Free T4 1.14, and the Free T3 0.19. Here the TSH was slightly elevated, (this is important because TSH above 2.0 is associated with developing osteoporosis) the Free T4 was fine, but the Free T3 was far too low, resulting in a ratio of approximately 0.17 or 17 percent. This accounted for her feeling sluggish and unrested after sleep.

Carol was functionally hypothyroid. Since Carol's T4 was normal and the T3 was too low, I treated her with Cytomel (T3) at a dosage of 12.5 mcgs. in the morning. Within four days, Carol was feeling improvement in her energy levels. After two weeks, her energy level was better than it had been in years. After nine months, her system "kicked in," and she was able to come off of the thyroid hormone completely.

Bob would wake up tired, had put on weight, was not motivated, and was very constipated. His TSH was 1.8, Free T4 was 0.86, Free T3 was 0.41 and his ratio was 0.48, or 48 percent. Bob's problem was iodine deficiency. His Free T4 was very low, but Free T3 was normal. When Bob was treated with Kelp tablets, his thyroid symptoms subsided, energy levels improved, and he was no longer constipated.

Betty was 52 years old and tired all of the time. She was constipated and bothered by dry, splitting nails and scaly skin. Her blood test showed a TSH of 2.8, Free T4 of 1.2, and Free T3 of 0.42. All of her numbers were within normal limits. She had an excellent ratio with good conversion, but her TSH was slightly elevated. Since Betty had the symptoms of hypothyroidism and slight elevation of TSH, she was treated with low-dose T4. Within two weeks, she was feeling much improved.

Brenda also exhibited symptoms of low thyroid. Her TSH was 3.0, Free T4 borderline low at 0.98, and Free T3 was 0.20, which means a low conversion of 20% and low T4 production. She responded well to Armour Thyroid.

Mary, a 36-year-old flight attendant, suffered from fatigue, muscle aches, and brain fog. She was unable to concentrate and focus. She would forget where she left things or where she was going. She thought maybe it was due to her job. She took a vacation, but nothing changed. Mary tried exercising and different diets to no avail. She was an attractive young woman with good muscle tone, but her skin was slightly dry, and her nails were a bit soft. She admitted being a little constipated, and she stated over and over again that no matter how well she slept she still woke up tired. When she was physically active, she would be fine for awhile, but she stopped, she dropped." She tended to be somewhat cold and needed a sweater even indoors. Mary had a blood test for thyroid and was told that everything was within normal limits and that no treatment was necessary. However, when I evaluated the tests, I saw that for her they were clearly abnormal. This is a common error because the range that is normal is quite broad and what is normal for one person may be abnormal for another. After taking Armour Thyroid for two weeks, her fatigue lifted, her bowels moved, her mood improved, she woke up refreshed, and she no longer suffered from brain fog.

Treatment

Fortunately, hypothyroidism is easily corrected and does not necessarily require treatment for the rest of your life. Once the diagnosis is made and you're prescribed the right thyroid hormone, you should see results within one to two weeks. The key to prescribing thyroid medications properly is to understand the problem thoroughly.

Popular Thyroid Medications

There are essentially three forms of thyroid medication: T4, T3, and a combination of T4 and T3.

Levothyroxine, also known as T4 (Levothyroid, Synthroid, Levoxyl or Unithroid)
These medications can be valuable in treating patients with a low T4 output, especially if the patient's T4/T3 ratio is appropriate. These are unstable compounds of thyroid and must be kept refrigerated. They are not good after 6 months.

Triiodothyronine or Liothyronine; or T3 (also known as Cytomel)
Cytomel is a form of pure T3 that is taken to correct an imbalance of the T4 to T3 ratio. If one has too much T4 and not enough T3, one can benefit from taking Cytomel.

Combination Thyroid Preparations
Armour Thyroid was the original thyroid supplement. It is an extract of pig thyroid glands. The glands have been desiccated, sterilized, standardized, and encapsulated for human consumption. This is one of the few instances where an animal source of hormones is identical to human hormones and directly applicable. Armour Thyroid is the most stable form of thyroid. It is especially valuable for people who have low T4 and a poor conversion of T4 to T3. The Broda Barnes Foundation promotes the use of Armour Thyroid as the best way to regulate hypothyroidism. They feel that it is the safest, the best tested, and the most natural form of thyroid with the highest rate of success.

Thyrolair is a synthetic combination of T4 and T3 with identical ratios to Armour Thyroid. Thyrolair, however, lacks other agents found in the glandular extract, such as Calcitonin, T2, and the stabilizing components of the gland that keep the thyroid active longer and not requiring refrigeration. Thyrolair is a good alternative for people who need both T4 and T3 but do not wish to take the glandular product. In my experience, I have found Armour Thyroid superior to Thyrolair in terms of people's response to the treatment.

Combining Products

In complicated cases, I have had to combine products to customize a blend that would best suit the patient. All of the thyroid products are compatible, and they can all be taken at the same time if need be. They should always be taken first thing in the morning on an empty stomach because food, especially minerals, can block absorption.

Evaluate Your Test Results

Use the following chart as a guide for determining which thyroid medication you need.

Problem	Solution
Elevated TSH, low T4, and low T3. T3 to T4 ratio is good (0.30-0.35).	T4
Elevated TSH, normal-to-somewhat-elevated T4, and low T3; i.e., low ratio.	Cytomel
Normal TSH, low T4, low T3 and low ratio.	Armour Thyroid or Iodine
Normal TSH, normal T3, normal T4, and normal ratio	Problem is not hypothyroidism. Search for other causes of the patient's symptoms.

Too Much Thyroid Hormone?

If you are taking too much thyroid medication, you may experience insomnia, palpitations, irritability, agitation, weight loss, and tremors. These side effects subside in one week if you reduce your dosage. Rarely, if ever, will there be any serious complications from a thyroid medication dosage that is too high if it is managed in a timely fashion.

Self-Help Measures

The Foods You Eat

The foods you eat can help or hinder your thyroid. Knowing which foods to emphasize or eliminate in your diet will help you protect your thyroid gland.

Nutrients That Support Your Thyroid

Nutrients that support the thyroid gland include iodine, zinc, vitamin A, vitamin E, the B vitamins, and Tyrosine.

Nutrient	Source
Iodine	Cod, sea bass, haddock, perch, Swiss chard, turnip greens, garlic, watercress, pineapples, pears, artichokes, citrus fruit, and egg yolks
	Kelp and other sea vegetables such as kombu, hijiki, nori, arame, sea palm, bladderwack, wakame, dulse, and Irish Moss
Zinc	Lamb, liver, steak, garlic, ginger root, brazil nuts, pumpkin seeds, oysters, eggs, sardines, oats, crab, almonds, and chicken
Vitamin A and Beta Carotene	Orange-colored fruits and vegetables, green leafy vegetables, liver, spinach, asparagus, milk, and fish liver oil
Vitamin E	Olive oil, leafy greens, whole grain cereals, avocado, fresh nuts, sunflower seeds, wheat germ, and eggs
B Vitamins	Colored fruits and vegetables, green leafy vegetables, bananas, oily fish, meat, eggs and fish oil
Selenium	Onions, milk, eggs, kelp, mushrooms, and garlic
L-Tyrosine	An amino acid produced from phenylalanine. which is found in most protein sources. Diets low in protein or with slow conversion of phenylalanine to L-Tyrosine may require supplemental L-Tyrosine

Foods That Suppress Your Thyroid
Foods that suppress the thyroid gland are called goitrogenic foods.

Food	Source
Raw foods that interfere with iodine uptake (cooked is fine)	Kale, cabbage, cauliflower, broccoli, kohlrabi, turnips, rutabagas, rapeseed, mustard, cassava, lima beans, linseed, peanuts, soybeans, and millet
Fluoride	Fluoridated drinking water, black tea, and fluoride drops

The Iodine Story

Regions vary in their soil content of trace minerals and nutrients. This gives unique flavor and character to the produce grown in those particular regions. The Midwest has excellent fertile soil, except that it is lacking in iodine. Produce grown in the Midwest is, therefore, generally low in iodine. Since many people eating local produce tended to develop an iodine deficiency, the Midwest became known as the Goiter Belt. A goiter is an enlarged thyroid gland that occurs when there is a deficiency of iodine in the diet. People with goiters looks like they have a large lump in their throat.

When the brain recognizes the need for more thyroid hormone, it sends out TSH to the thyroid gland to produce more hormone. If the thyroid gland is unable to produce more thyroid hormone because of lack of iodine, the brain gets a signal that there is not enough iodine and produces more TSH. This stimulates the thyroid even more, and the vicious cycle causes the thyroid gland to enlarge and form a goiter.

In an effort to control goiter, especially in the Midwest, scientists realized that people had to be supplemented with iodine. The only way they could be assured of getting adequate iodine into people in a form that could be easily stored was to put iodine into salt. Iodized salt became the vehicle to supplement the diet with iodine.

Although iodized salt offers a solution as an iodine supplement for many people in this country, the advent of salt-restricted diets for hypertension and heart disease is now thought to be a major cause of hypothyroidism, especially in the elderly. This is especially striking because there is an epidemic of hypothyroidism in this country that is for the most part undetected. Hypothyroidism can masquerade as depression or just old age.

Many people choose to use natural sea salt. Although sea salt contains many other elements, it is not a good source of iodine. If you use a sea salt or are on a salt-free diet and experience symptoms of hypothyroidism, you should be checked for iodine deficiency.

Supplements

There are three primary supplements that encourage thyroid hormone development. The first one obviously is iodine, the second is zinc, and the third is L-tyrosine.

Iodine

Iodine supplements come in many forms. The goal is to get 150 mcg of iodine per day in the diet, and for pregnant and nursing women, 200 mcg per day. Too little iodine can result in hypothyroidism and may not be recognizable for quite some time because the body can store enough iodine to fortify the thyroid gland for up to a year. Excess ingestion of iodine will not have any serious effects over the short term. However, prolonged excesses of iodine in doses of 1,000 mcg per day can overstimulate or even shut down the thyroid gland.

Kelp

Kelp is an easy way to obtain iodine in the form of a supplement. Kelp is a seaweed that is readily available in most health food stores in tablets or capsules. Usually one or two per day is all that is needed.

Zinc

Zinc is a critical mineral for the support of the thyroid gland. It should always be taken in balance with copper in a ratio of 15 to 1. Since the average zinc requirement for thyroid health would be 30 mg. of zinc, it would require a balance of 2 mg. of copper.

L-Tyrosine
L-Tyrosine is a valuable amino acid that has many functions. One important function is its use as a building block for thyroid hormone. Deficiencies of L-tyrosine in the diet can result in deficiencies of thyroid hormone. This is a very safe amino acid to ingest. 3,000 mg. is considered therapeutic. It should be taken in divided doses twice a day.

Exercise

Exercise enhances the function of every organ of the body. It helps the thyroid gland function by stimulating the production of thyroid hormone. Exercise improves metabolism, digestion and circulation, elevates the mood, and alleviates stress. Exercise should be fun, safe, done on a regular basis, and be somewhat aerobic.

Resources

Sea Vegetables

Packaged sea vegetables are available in natural food stores and Asian markets around the country. In the Western diet, they may be added to soups, stews, salads or baked potatoes.

Mail Order Sources
If you cannot find a store in your area that sells sea vegetables, the following mail order sources will ship vegetables:
Sea Vegetable Company
P.O. Box 1256
Mendocino, CA 95460
(707) 937-2050
Contact: Eleanor and John Lewallen

Natural Lifestyle Supplies
16 Lookout Drive
Asheville, NC 28804
(800) 752-2775
www.natural-lifestyle.com

Contact: Tom, tom@natural-lifestyle.com
Sells ground seaweed in a vegicap ($19.95, 100 per bottle) for people who want the benefits of seaweed but don't want to add it to their food.

Western Isles
P.O. Box 3577
London NW2 1LQ
Great Britain

CHAPTER 5

Sex Hormones and the Brain

Hormones are chemical messengers that are sent through the bloodstream to tell the cells how to function. Produced in very small amounts by a gland in one part of the body, they have profound effects on organs and tissues in other parts of the body.

The sex hormones: testosterone, estrogen, progesterone, and dehydroepiandrosterone (DHEA) are formed from testicular, ovarian, or adrenocortical tissues and affect the development of both primary sexual characteristics (i.e., the genitals), and secondary characteristics—those characteristics that make one appear masculine or feminine, such as broadness of shoulders, muscle mass, hips, breasts, voice, distribution of hair, and brain function.

Although political correctness has tried to abolish common sense and empirical evidence, hormonal differences in men and women do create differences in how their brains function. Women tend to excel in verbal fluency, fine motor coordination, memory for word lists, object location, and perceptual speed. Men, however, tend to excel in spatial skills, target-directed motor skills, and mathematical reasoning.

Testosterone and the Brain

Testosterone has profound effects on the brain. In the 2001 edition of *Principles and Practices of Endocrinology and Metabolism,* the following characteristics of testosterone were delineated:

- Improves energy levels
- Elevates mood
- Gives overall feeling of well-being

- Increases physical strength
- Improves sexual drive (libido)
- Improves motivation and initiative
- Improves perception of spatial relationships
- Improves verbal memory
- Improves sleep quality

Testosterone for Pain

Testosterone is very useful for the treatment of chronic pain. When testosterone levels are adequate, muscles are stronger, tissues are more resilient, the mood is elevated, and chronic pain frequently goes away. Other benefits include:

- Faster healing of fractures
- Lower blood sugar in diabetics
- Improved heart function
- Improved circulation
- Increased stability of the body

Testosterone in Men

In men, testosterone levels are diagnosed through symptoms, as well as by blood tests. Symptoms of inadequate testosterone include decreases in:

- Muscle mass
- Libido
- Enthusiasm
- Motivation
- Blood count
- Facial hair
- Appetite
- Mood (depression)

Addition symptoms include:
- Poor memory
- Heart disease
- Increased fat around the abdomen

Typically, testosterone levels in men at the age of 45 are half of what they were at the age of 25. Men can sometimes have normal levels of testosterone in their blood but still have all of the symptoms of low testosterone because their body craves more for optimal function. Testosterone deficiency is common in diabetics, particularly type 2 (non-insulin-dependent diabetics) as well as in those suffering from Syndrome X, characterized by high blood pressure, high cholesterol levels, low testosterone, and elevated blood sugar in the presence of elevated insulin.

Testosterone Treatment for Men

Andropause, or male menopause, is a normal part of aging. The profound effect that low levels of testosterone have on men undergoing andropause cannot be overstated. Any man over the age of 40, especially if he has undergone a shock or a lot of stress and is experiencing depression, sadness, lack of motivation, irritability, or mood changes, is most probably going through andropause and is a prime candidate for testosterone replacement therapy. For these men, recovery without testosterone replacement therapy is unlikely. Men who are undergoing andropause will have a dramatic relief of their symptoms, oftentimes within days after their first injection of testosterone. Some men require three doses of testosterone by injection until the right dose is achieved and their symptoms are alleviated.

Treating Testosterone Deficiency

There are two ways to treat testosterone deficiency in men.

Stimulate the body to produce its own testosterone with Human Chorionic Gonatropin (HCG)
HCG stimulates testosterone production in the testicles. Although HCG cannot stimulate the body to produce large amounts of testosterone, it can give it a bit of a boost, which may be all that is needed to improve function. Treatment is accomplished through injection twice a week. If you can give yourself an injection at home, you can safely stimulate your own body to produce testosterone. However, since many people have a hard time giving themselves a shot, HCG may not be an option for them.

Supplement the Body with Testosterone
The following forms of testosterone may be administered to increase the level of testosterone in a man's body:

Pellets are produced in the shape of small cylinders that hold testosterone in a matrix so that it dissolves over time. In most men, standard pellets last between six and ten weeks whereas the long-acting pellets last between four and six months before they need to be replaced. Placement is usually in the area of the hip or the lower abdomen under the skin and the procedure takes approximately five minutes. Pellets are very safe, effective, long-lasting, painless, and most important of all, convenient. Frequency of administration is determined by how fast the body metabolizes the testosterone. This is determined by blood tests taken once a month or by the patient's symptoms. Once the pattern has been established, blood tests no longer need to be repeated.

Oral (pills) contain Methyltestosterone and are not recommended because they have been shown to cause liver damage and liver cancer.

Creams and Topical Forms of testosterone are not a good option because they tend to convert to estrogen. Excess estrogen serves only to compound the problem of inadequate levels of testosterone. If a man does decide to take topical testosterone, he may need to take an aromatase inhibitor to block the conversion of testosterone to estrogen. (See section on Aromatase.)

Testosterone via Injection may be given every two weeks in doses that range from 100 to 500 mg. The preferred preparation of testosterone is Testosterone Cypionate.

Aromatase

Some men have an increased level of aromatase, which is an enzyme that rapidly converts testosterone into estrogen. The result is that testosterone has a feminizing effect on the man. By inhibiting aromatase, the testosterone levels can be increased and estrogen levels decreased without supplemental testosterone. Fat has high levels of aromatase and, therefore, obese men may not be able to experience the benefit of taking testosterone because the fat is converting the testosterone into estrogen.

Aromatase inhibitors come in two forms, natural and synthetic. The natural aromatase inhibitors, Diindolymethane (DIM) and Indol-3-Carbinol (I-3-C), are derived from cruciferous vegetables. They are not as potent as the synthetic aromatase inhibitors—Anastrozole (Arimidex), Exemestane (Aromasin), and Trozole (Famara)—but they are far less toxic and less expensive.

Testing for Testosterone Deficiency

Testing for testosterone is accomplished with a blood or saliva test. Testing is best done either before 10:00 a.m., when testosterone levels are at their highest, or after 4:00 p.m. when levels are at their lowest.

When testing for testosterone, one must test for the following:

Total Testosterone

Total testosterone reflects how much testosterone is in the blood.

Free Testosterone

Free testosterone reflects how much of the total testosterone is available for use. One can have a normal and even high level of total testosterone but a low level of free, meaning that the hormone is not available to be used by the cells.

Prostate Specific Antigen (PSA)

An evaluation for prostate cancer is critical in men who are considering testosterone therapy. Although testosterone will NOT cause prostate cancer, it can make it worse. PSA levels can be elevated if prostate cancer is present, but they can also be due to an infection or inflammation of the prostate. Careful monitoring of the PSA is critical during a course of testosterone therapy.

Estradiol

Estradiol is a metabolite of testosterone. Elevated levels of estradiol in men can complicate testosterone replacement therapy. If a man has a tendency to have elevated levels of estradiol, he must receive an aromatase blocker; otherwise, not only will the testosterone treatments not be as effective as they could be, but it may have a reverse effect because of the elevated level of estrogen.

DHEA-S

DHEA-S is the more stable form of DHEA found in the body. It is important for two reasons. It converts to testosterone in women, and in both men and women it is found to play a significant role in brain function, mood, and immune-system functioning.

Testosterone in Women

Although testosterone is considered to be a male hormone, women also need testosterone, although in much lower doses than men. There are two prominent indications that a woman may be low in testosterone. They are:

- A low libido (poor sex drive)
- Osteoporosis

Other signs of low testosterone levels include:

- Poor healing
- Thin, fragile skin
- Scant pubic hair
- Poor coordination
- Weakness
- Depression
- Lack of motivation

Women who are supplemented with appropriate levels of testosterone experience an increase of:

- Strength and agility
- Sense of well-being
- Libido
- Prevention and reversal of osteoporosis
- Improved spatial relationship

DHEA in Women

In women (but not in men), DHEA serves as a precursor (a building block) from which testosterone is formed. Many women can take DHEA and bring testosterone levels up to an acceptable range without having to worry about testosterone injections, pellets, or creams. The effects of taking the DHEA are usually felt within six to eight weeks.

When replacing DHEA or testosterone in women, one must be very careful to make sure that adequate levels of estrogen and progesterone are also given at the same time to avoid any unwanted side effects.

Side Effects of Testosterone Treatment in Women

It is very important that women who take supplemental testosterone work with their doctor to make sure that all of their hormones are in balance. Any amount of testosterone without adequate levels of estrogen will promote unwanted hair growth, deepening of the voice, acne, and male pattern baldness. Balancing hormones frequently takes time, and until the hormones are balanced, some women may experience menstrual irregularities and/or spotting. Should a woman experience any of these side effects, she need not worry, as they are easily reversed once a proper balance has been obtained. Women experiencing hair growth problems can take a medication called Spironolactone along with the testosterone to prevent unwanted facial hair.

Which Women Should Take Testosterone?

Symptoms of low testosterone usually correspond with menopause; however, many women taking birth control pills experience the symptoms of low testosterone as well. There is new evidence that the birth control pill, in addition to suppressing estrogen and progesterone production, also suppresses testosterone production. Hence, many younger women will experience problems with low testosterone.

Case Study: Tara

Tara, a very athletic 26-year old woman, did a well-rehearsed flip at a friend's wedding forgetting that she was wearing high heels and not sneakers. When she landed, she broke her foot. Even after the cast removal and physical therapy, she had chronic, disabling pain for nine months before I saw her. Blood tests showed she had low testosterone levels due to the fact that she was taking birth control pills. After receiving testosterone treatments for two weeks, her fracture began healing and by eight weeks was completely healed.

Studies have shown that young women who have a sudden decrease in testosterone are far more susceptible to developing breast cancer. Since aromatase inhibitors increase levels of testosterone by preventing the conversion of testosterone into estrogen, it is a useful medication in the treatment and prevention of breast cancer.

Contraindications of Testosterone in Women

A word of caution: Testosterone should never be given to a woman who is pregnant, who is trying to become pregnant, or who could become pregnant. A female fetus could experience many problems with a higher-than-normal level of testosterone and can undergo virilization.

Treatment of Testosterone Deficiency in Women

Testosterone therapy options for women include a topical cream, injection, pellets, or suppository.

Testosterone Cream

Testosterone cream must be applied topically every night by smearing the prescribed dose over the largest possible area of skin. The more pores you cover, the more the cream will be absorbed.

Testosterone Patch

A more convenient form of applying the cream is using the testosterone patch. The problem with the patches is that they frequently cause skin irritation and some of them contain a form of testosterone called Methyltestosterone which can be toxic to the liver. Patches tend to be two to five times more expensive than the cream.

Testosterone Injections

Many women prefer injections because they last two to four weeks. The recommended dose is 25 to 100 mg. Injections keep a steady level of testosterone in the body and seems to have a more beneficial effect on brain function and memory enhancement than do topical forms.

Pellets

Pellets are very convenient and economical for women because they can last up to six months.

Suppositories

Testosterone is efficiently absorbed in the form of a suppository that can be inserted rectally or vaginally. This needs to be done nightly or every other night, depending on how the testosterone is being metabolized.

Estrogen and the Brain

Natural estrogen enhances the function of the brain cells that allow enhancement of memory in women. This is accomplished through several mechanisms:

Improved Blood Flow to the Brain

Estrogen improves blood flow to the brain by as much as 30 percent.

Enhancing Brain Cell Activity

By enhancing brain cell activity, estrogen also improves memory and cognition, postural stability, balance, movement, and fine motor skills. It elevates mood and protects the brain from damage due to injury and neuro-degenerative diseases. Estrogen enhances verbal abilities, as well as perceptual speed and accuracy, and slows the aging process of the brain.

Serotonin Availability

Estrogen also has an antidepressant effect on the brain by making serotonin more available to the brain cells themselves. Women who take antidepressants such as the SSRIs (Zoloft, Prozac, Paxil, etc.) fare better if they are also taking estrogen or if they already have adequate estrogen.

Nerve Growth

Estrogen is also a neuro-protective hormone because of its ability to stimulate a nerve growth factor, and it protects the brain from damage caused by toxic exposure.

Estrogen is divided into three forms:

Estrone (E1)—a potent form of estrogen whose primary function is to serve as a reservoir for Estradiol. Ogen is Estrone's pharmaceutical name.

Estradiol (E2)—the primary form of estrogen that has the strongest estrogen-related effects on the body. Estrace is Estradiol's pharmaceutical name.

Estriol (E3)—the weakest form of estrogen, it is known for its anti-cancer effects. It serves as a reservoir for Estradiol. Estriol is not available as a pharmaceutical prescription. It is, however, available through a compounding pharmacist.

Appropriate balance of the estrogens allows for optimal benefit with the minimal dose and lowest cost. There are two basic combinations: Biest and Triest. Biest is 80% Estriol and 20% Estradiol. Triest is 80% Estriol, 10% Estradiol, and 10% Estrone.

Facts related to Estrogen and Memory

As early as 1954, estrogen replacement therapy was shown to improve cognition in elderly post-menopausal women, and improvements were noted in comprehension, language, naming, and math skills. Significant findings include:

Estradiol Levels in Women with Alzheimer's
Estradiol levels are significantly lower in post-menopausal women with Alzheimer's compared to women in the same age group who are not suffering from Alzheimer's. These neurophysiological effects of estrogen on the

brain may explain the correlation of estrogen deficiency with cognitive impairment in the development of Alzheimer's-type dementia.

Estrogen Treatment Has a Direct Effect on Cognitive Function
Well-designed studies have shown that estrogen treatment has a direct benefit on discreet cognitive functions including paragraph recall and immediate and delayed associate learning. This may be due to the fact that estrogen improves cerebral blood flow in women. It has also been shown to improve EEG performance.

Estrogen and Menopause

Estrogen is primarily known for its feminizing effects on women. It increases the blood flow and proliferation of the endometrium (the lining of the uterus) in preparation to receive a fertilized egg. It also is important for maintaining calcium in the bones and lubrication of the vagina.

Estrogen production in some women actually increases with menopause. This increase, combined with a woman's natural loss of progesterone, creates a situation called *estrogen dominance.* Interestingly, in those women whose estrogen levels continue to be normal after menopause, their cognitive and emotional changes are primarily due to the loss of progesterone. Most women however, do experience a loss of estrogen production during menopause and pre-menopause and suffer from mood changes, as well as loss of proper thought pattern and memory.

Surgical Menopause

Women who have undergone a total hysterectomy will lose their ability to produce the hormones progesterone and estrogen. Hence, they commonly suffer from changes in mood, memory, and cognition (thinking). They generally respond well when given supplemental doses of appropriate estrogens and progesterone.

Human Identical Hormones

When replacing estrogen, it is best to use natural estrogens that are identical to human estrogens to avoid the side effects of synthetic hormones.

When taking natural hormone replacement therapy, the skin becomes softer and less dry, women appear more youthful, facial hair sometimes disappears and the normal shape of a woman's body can return. Women report feeling more feminine and sexier.

Synthetic Estrogens

Synthetic estrogens are non-human compatible compounds with some estrogen-like activity. Ethinyl Estradiol is frequently used in birth control pills because it has a very high potency and is able to shut down the reproductive system.

The second most common form, Premarin, is made from horse estrogen. Premarin stands for PREgnant MARre urINe. Premarin, however, is not estrogen—it is a group of horse hormones called *equilins.* The side effects of Premarin include: blood clots, heart disease, strokes, depression, senility, cancer, weight gain, and mood changes.

Prescribing Estrogen

The primary sign that women are deficient in estrogen is vaginal dryness. Women can have a thick, milky-white vaginal discharge and still be low on estrogen because the discharge is due to irritation of the vaginal wall. A blood test or saliva test for hormone levels is necessary to diagnose low hormone levels and to provide information about the appropriate replacement therapy. Proper natural hormone replacement therapy will usually alleviate symptoms within one or two weeks. Additional benefits of estrogen replacement include mood enhancement, improved memory, and the elimination of hot flashes.

Estrogen can be taken in four forms:

Pill

When taking estrogen orally, one should always take it with food in the morning. Some women may need to take it twice a day. Pills tend to have a high peak but a shorter half-life. This means that the pill form is absorbed faster but metabolized more quickly.

Cream

Creams have a longer lasting effect without the profound peaking of blood levels and rapid drop off that can occur with an oral form, but many women find it difficult to remember to apply the cream daily.

Suppository

Many women prefer vaginal suppositories because they also improve vaginal lubrication.

Pellets

Pellets inserted under the skin can last between two to six months and provide a continuous level of estrogen to the body. This is the preferred method for women who have difficulty taking medication on a regular basis; however, it may cause spotting.

The dose for pills, cream, and suppositories is 2.5 to 5.0 mg. given once or twice a day. The subdermal pellets are given in doses of 50 to 100 mg.

Progesterone's Role in Menstruation

Progesterone's job is to limit proliferation of the endometrium and to maintain integrity of breast and uterine tissues. During a woman's cycle, a drop in the progesterone level occurs at the end of the cycle prior to the onset of bleeding. This drop usually takes a few days at which time PMS (pre-menstrual syndrome) may occur.

Progesterone's Role in Bone Density and Brain Health

Progesterone, known as "the other female hormone," facilitates uptake of estrogen into the brain.

As soon as the menstrual flow begins, PMS symptoms tend to ease. When estrogen levels begin to rise, menstrual flow ceases. The endometrium, i.e., the lining of the uterus, begins to grow and proliferate. Progesterone is then secreted to modulate the effect of estrogens on the uterus so that the endometrium does not grow out of balance. It also keeps the endometrium from discharging too soon. Therefore, it can delay the onset of the menstrual cycle.

Progesterone is also critical in maintaining bone density even when estrogen levels are adequate. In addition, progesterone has been shown to induce myelination of axons (fixing the insulation around the nerve cells) after nerves have been damaged. In women and men, progesterone plays a role in recovery from brain injury. Women and men who have suffered brain injury recover faster if they have high levels of progesterone.

Advantages of Taking Human Identical Progesterone

- Enhances focus
- Elevates the mood
- Calms the nervous system
- Improves bone density
- Improves memory
- Prevents breast and uterine cancer
- Decreases fluid retention
- Regulates blood pressure
- Enhances recovery of the brain from trauma such as concussions
- Enhances sleep quality

GABA Receptors and Progesterone's Calming Effect

The cells of the brain have receptors that induce a calming effect on nerve activity. These receptors are called GABA (gamma amino butyric acid) receptors. There are two GABA receptors: GABA A and GABA B. Anything that stimulates a GABA receptor will cause a calming effect on the nervous system. Progesterone binds to GABA A. Benzodiazepines (for example, Valium) bind to GABA B. Both progesterone and benzodiazepines will bind (or stimulate) the GABA receptors of the brain cells, resulting in a calming effect. Studies have shown that low levels of progesterone can result in high levels of anxiety. Therefore, women who are pre- or post-menopausal and are experiencing anxiety and mood changes will most likely benefit from taking supplemental progesterone rather than Valium.

Women also experience mood changes associated with low levels of progesterone during post-partum depression. Proper supplementation with progesterone can often alleviate post-partum depression. *(Note:* Post-partum depression may also be due to thyroid. See chapter on thyroid.)

Pharmaceutical Progesterone

There are essentially six progesterone substitutes. Five are used primarily for birth control pills, and the sixth is primarily for post-menopausal symptoms. The most commonly prescribed substitute for progesterone for post-menopausal women is Medroxyprogesterone which is also known as Provera. It is the prototype of all of the progesterone substitutes. As a group, all of the variations of progesterone are called progestins. Natural progesterone is also in the category of progestins, but it is the only one that can be called progesterone. This is an important distinction, because progestins are defined as a group of hormones which have progestational effects on the uterine lining. Progestins limit the growth of the lining of the uterus and oppose the stimulation by estrogens. This is basically where the similarity between progestins and progesterone stops.

Progestins

Synthetic progestins are generally far more potent than progesterone in regard to the effect on the uterus and the body in general. For example, Medroxyprogesterone (Provera) is 20 times stronger than progesterone and is not metabolized by the liver in the same way as progesterone. This, however, is not an accident—this is by design.

Pharmaceutical companies were faced with a dilemma. Women going through menopause needed hormone replacement therapy. Natural hormones are not patentable however, and therefore are not profitable for the drug companies. Also, hormones are generally metabolized by the liver. By altering the hormone to block the breakdown by the liver, they were able to sustain its action and increase its potency. In addition, the altered hormones could now be patented, making them profitable for the drug companies. They also wanted to create a hormone which was inexpensive to manufacture. Medroxyprogesterone solved these problems because it was both inexpensive to manufacture and patentable.

Side Effects of Synthetic Progestins

- Fluid retention
- Increased incidence of breast and uterine cancer
- Increased incidence of heart disease and strokes
- Increased agitation and irritability
- Blocking the effectiveness of estrogen on the brain, thereby causing memory loss
- Interfering with sleep, which further exacerbates mood changes

In an article by L.J. Melton entitled *"Sex and the Brain,"* Melton describes how Provera blocks the beneficial effects of estrogen on the brain. He further notes that rather than create a feeling of calm, clarity, and focus, the way that progesterone does, Provera decreases brain function, thereby causing brain fog.

Despite Provera's detrimental side effects that have been well known for over 20 years, it remains the most common form of progesterone prescribed for women during menopause. Many practitioners believe Provera's popularity is due to aggressive marketing by drug companies that convince physicians that Provera is progesterone. Remember, Provera is not progesterone.

Progesterone Supplementation

Progesterone can be taken by injection, pills, cream, or pellets.

Injection

Injected natural progesterone can have beneficial effects that last from two to four weeks. However, levels can drop off relatively rapidly after that.

Depo-Provera has been used for many years as a means of birth control and also as a means of controlling uterine bleeding. It is a high-dose injection of Medroxyprogesterone (see above) that lasts up to six months and will stop a woman from having her period. However, because of the large number of side effects, it is not recommended except in extreme cases.

Pills

Progesterone is safe to take orally. Micronized progesterone, which blocks the rapid uptake and metabolism by the liver allowing longer duration of effect, is now available. Micronized progesterone is best taken with meals, as food enhances uptake. Progesterone taken with the evening meal enhances sleep quality, calms the nerves, and can stabilize mood in the morning upon awakening. A word of caution: Micronized progesterone, available as a prescription in a product called Prometrium, contains peanut oil. Women who are allergic to peanuts should avoid this product and instead have the product compounded by a compounding pharmacist.

The standard dose of progesterone is 100 to 400 mg. taken once or twice a day with food.

Cream

Applying progesterone topically is an option. The cream should be applied every night, usually at bedtime. It has a longer duration of action than does the oral preparation of progesterone. The downside is that many women find it difficult to remember to apply the cream every night.

The standard dose is 100 to 200 mg. When applying the cream, cover as large an area of your skin as possible. Remember, the more pores you cover, the more medicine will be absorbed.

Suppositories

Vaginal or rectal suppositories are probably the most efficient means of absorbing progesterone into the body. The dose varies from 50 to 200 mg. every one to three days.

Pellets

Progesterone pellets have the longest duration of action of any of the preparations of natural progesterone lasting from two to six months before they need to be replaced. It is the preferred method for women who have a hard time taking medications on a regular basis. The downside is that it can cause spotting.

Prempro

On July 9, 2002, an agency of the Federal Government and part of the National Institutes of Health halted a major clinical trial of the risks and benefits of hormone replacement therapy involving a drug called Prempro. Manufactured by Wyeth Laboratories, Prempro is a combination pill of Premarin and Provera that was found to increase the risk of breast cancer, heart attack, stroke, blood clots, and pulmonary embolism.

The shutdown of the clinical trial angered the more than 16 million women who were taking Prempro and several class action lawsuits were filed. The warnings that were issued became a wake-up call to doctors concerning synthetic drugs. (Note: The American College for Advancement in Medicine listed in the Resources section can help you find a doctor or nurse practitioner who can prescribe bio-identical hormones.)

The sad truth is that this information has been known for approximately 30 years. I am grateful for the honesty of the researchers who did that study and reported the results, while at the same time I'm frustrated that the scientific community has suppressed this information for so many years. Physicians who use bio-identical, natural hormones have been persecuted by the medical establishment when they were simply practicing good medicine and researching their products before prescribing them.

Case Study: Susan

Susan was married for 20 years, loved her husband and enjoyed her kids. Now that her kids were older, she had more time to do the things that she had always wanted to do. Unfortunately, she found that she had no desire to go back to school or begin anything new. She was just not motivated. Her lack of enthusiasm also affected her relationship with her husband. Although she loved her husband, her libido was gone. She was forgetful, and learning new things was difficult. She was worried that perhaps she might be becoming senile.

Susan knew she was going through menopause, as her periods were becoming more and more irregular. Her doctor told her that as long as she was having periods her hormones were still working and not to worry.

Still, she felt that something was not quite right and came in for an evaluation. Blood tests revealed that she had low testosterone, low DHEA, and low progesterone. Her estrogen levels, however, were normal.

When I put her on the appropriate hormones, Susan noticed dramatic changes within just a few weeks. Her memory improved, she was sleeping better, her moods were elevated, libido returned, she felt more enthusiastic, and she had a desire to return to school. This 48-year-old female now felt as strong, sharp, and sexy as she did when she was 25 years old.

Resources

Trade Secrets: A Moyers Report

2001, PBS
Trade Secrets: A Moyers Report is an investigation of the history of the chemical revolution and the companies that drove it—and how companies worked to withhold vital information about the risks from workers, the government, and the public. Journalist Bill Moyers and producer Sherry Jones rely on an archive of documents that the public was never meant to see—documents that reveal the industry's early knowledge that some chemicals could pose dangers to human health and were not disclosed at the time. www.pbs.org/tradesecrets

John E. Lee, M.D.

Known for his 1996 book, *What Your Doctor May Not Tell You about Menopause* and his 1999 book, *What Your Doctor May Not Tell You about Premenopause,* John Lee also publishes a medical newsletter:

The John R. Lee M.D. Medical Letter
P.O. Box 84900 Phoenix, AZ 95071
info@johnleemd.com (800) 528-0559

American College for Advancement in Medicine

(800) 532-3688

Publishes *Natural Answers for Women's Health Questions* and acts as a resource for locating a doctor or nurse practitioner who can prescribe bio-identical hormones.

CHAPTER 6

Hypoglycemia

Brain cells rely primarily on glucose, a form of sugar, for energy. Without glucose, the brain cells do not work adequately, resulting in difficulty focusing, concentrating, and responding appropriately to stress. Therefore, low blood sugar, or hypoglycemia, can have a profound effect on one's state of alertness.

In 1995, Philip Felig and his colleagues wrote in the textbook *Endocrinology and Metabolism,* "Glucose is an obligate fuel for the brain. Even brief hypoglycemic episodes can cause profound dysfunction of the brain."

Symptoms of hypoglycemia include:

- Irritability
- Temper outbursts
- Anxiety
- Psychological disturbances
- Indecisiveness
- Headaches
- Concentration difficulties
- Depression
- Palpitations
- Perspiration
- Lassitude
- Prolonged fatigue
- Incoherent speech
- Hunger
- Convulsions

Regulating Blood Sugar

Your body only needs about 2 teaspoons of glucose (sugar) circulating at any one time. Since too much or too little sugar is so damaging to the body, the body is designed with very precise controls to regulate blood sugar levels.

There are basically two hormones involved in stabilizing blood glucose which is so crucial for optimal brain function—insulin and glucagon. When the pancreas senses elevated levels of glucose in the blood, it secretes insulin. Insulin drives down glucose in the blood by pushing glucose into the cells (that's why increased insulin is implicated in weight gain). When the pancreas senses a low level of glucose in the blood, it secretes glucagons, which raises glucose in the blood. Insulin and glucagon work together to maintain the optimal level of glucose in the blood for your brain to function well. If, however, the pancreas is overwhelmed with a sudden, enormous intake of sugar, for example, drinking a can of cola (which contains 8–10 teaspoons of sugar), the pancreas can overreact, secreting too much insulin causing blood sugar to plummet, which results in hypoglycemia. To prevent such strong fluctuations of blood sugar, adequate protein and fats with each meal will stimulate glucagon secretion and keep blood sugar more level, which will minimize cravings.

Types of Hypoglycemia

Blood sugar levels that are too low (hypoglycemia) or too high (diabetes) can cause numerous health problems. In normal circumstances, the body maintains a consistent level of blood sugar within a narrow range (80 to 110 mg/dl) through the coordination of several glands and hormones. When the body's blood sugar control mechanism is overactive, hypoglycemia is the result.

There are two types of hypoglycemia:

- Reactive hypoglycemia
- Fasting hypoglycemia

Reactive Hypoglycemia

Reactive hypoglycemia, the most common type, is characterized by low blood sugar symptoms two to five hours after eating a meal high in sugar or carbohydrates.

High glycemic foods, foods that are converted rapidly to glucose (sugar), cause a rapid rise in glucose levels in the blood (See Glycemic Index in this chapter). When this occurs, the body responds by secreting a hormone called insulin, which puts the sugar into the cells. A second hormone called glucagon regulates the glucose in the blood by counteracting the effect of insulin. In this manner, blood glucose levels remain within a certain range.

In people who have reactive hypoglycemia, a rapid rise of blood glucose after ingesting a high glycemic meal (see below) is followed by overreaction of the pancreas to secrete more insulin than is necessary. This high level of insulin causes a dramatic drop in the blood glucose levels before the person is able to secrete enough glucagon to modify this response. What follows is a hypoglycemic reaction in which blood sugar levels plummet within two to five hours.

Why Hypoglycemics Get Irritable

As blood sugar levels plummet, the adrenal glands detect a crisis. In an effort to stabilize blood glucose levels, they secrete adrenaline (i.e., epinephrine) causing the body to feel jittery, nervous, and hyperactive. This, in turn, sets up a red flag in which adrenal glands now secrete another hormone called cortisol. The brain, now on hyper-alert, may actually experience feelings of euphoria, but this does not last long before the crash occurs. Soon, one becomes incoherent, foggy, and apathetic, with a dramatic change of mood. These feelings may make a person panic and reach for some sugar to raise blood glucose levels starting the cycle all over again.

Fasting Hypoglycemia

Fasting hypoglycemia is the rarest and the most serious form of hypoglycemia. It refers to the existence of hypoglycemia symptoms that occur more than five hours after eating. In contrast, reactive hypoglycemics experience symptoms less than 5 hours after eating (usually within two to three hours after eating). Symptoms of *fasting hypoglycemia* will frequently present themselves in the middle of the night while a person is sleeping or in the morning upon awakening. For people who have *reactive hypoglycemia,* these are the times when blood sugar is most stable.

Causes of fasting hypoglycemia include:

Pancreatic Tumors (Insulinoma)
A growth on the pancreas will increase its size and also increase the amount of insulin produced.

Deficiencies in the Adrenal, Pituitary, or Thyroid Glands
All hormones in the body work interdependently to form a tapestry that should create a sense of health and well-being. Imbalances in any of the hormones in the endocrine system can result in low blood sugar, elevated thyroid, elevated epinephrine (adrenaline), low levels of glucagon, deficiencies of digestive enzymes, or too much cortisol.

Alcohol
In alcoholics, fasting hypoglycemia can result from liver damage.

Drugs
Drugs that may cause fasting hypoglycemia include:

Drug	Description
Quinine	A drug used to treat malaria and leg cramps
Quinidine	A drug used to treat heart rhythm irregularities
Salicylates	Aspirin-like drugs
Sulfa drugs	Antibiotic
Disopyr amide	Anti-arrhythmic heart medication.
Propoxyphene	A pain medication also known as Darvon or Darvocet
Haloperiodol	An antipsychotic drug
Pen tami dine	An antibiotic used in the treatment of AIDS
All Oral Hypoglycemics	Drugs used to lower blood sugar levels in Type II Diabetics can lower blood sugar levels too far, resulting in hypoglycemia

Important Note: Beta blockers such as Atenolol, Propranolol, Toprol, or Lopressor can mask the symptoms of hypoglycemia and should always be used with caution by diabetics, especially if they are taking insulin.

Insulin Dependent Diabetics

For those diabetics who are taking insulin to regulate their blood glucose, too much insulin will drive blood sugar down so low that it can cause severe hypoglycemia. This is an emergency. An overdose of insulin can cause a critical drop of glucose, causing diabetics to become lethargic, confused, and even have seizures and go into a coma. All diabetics taking insulin should be cautioned about the warning signs of overdose of insulin, and they should have a source of sugar with them at all times, should they overdose.

Adrenal Response to Low Blood Sugar Levels

When sugar levels reach a low point, the adrenal glands release a small amount of adrenaline, causing the liver to release glucose. In most people, the secretion of adrenaline will cause sugar levels to rise to normal levels. In people who have hypoglycemia, researchers have found that there may be a surge of sugar-mobilizing stress hormones.

Researchers at the University of Maryland, Johns Hopkins University, and the National Institutes of Health have identified an adrenaline/cortisol connection in people who have hypoglycemic symptoms three or four hours after eating a meal high in carbohydrates. At the bottom of the sugar curve, when blood sugar is at its lowest, people who are hypoglycemic experience a surge in adrenaline and cortisol. These surges of adrenaline and cortisol are the primary causes of the symptoms of hypoglycemia; i.e., anxiety, irritability, hyperreactive, crowded thinking, increased heart rate, nervousness, and sweating. In people with hypoglycemia, adrenaline levels increased by more than 1200 percent when blood sugar levels were at a low point. These same people also showed a distinct increase in cortisol. Both adrenaline and cortisol can produce symptoms associated with hypoglycemia.

Syndrome X

High sugar intake in the diet not only contributes to hypoglycemia, but it is also linked to heart disease, diabetes, and free radical stress from the oxidation of glucose. Glucose oxidizes much faster than fat. As a result, many scientists believe that excess sugar is far more dangerous than fat.

Excessive intake of sugar and carbohydrates has become so prevalent, that new terminology has evolved to describe a cluster of physiological problems that are largely due to sugar addiction. Syndrome X is a condition characterized by elevated insulin levels, elevated blood sugar levels, elevated blood pressure, elevated cholesterol, and obesity. Since insulin and blood sugar are both elevated at the same time, the brain does not know whether to stimulate the pancreas to produce more insulin to lower the sugar, or shut down the pancreas to lower the insulin. Usually, the pancreas is stimulated to produce more insulin.

Syndrome X and Testosterone

A common, but little known factor associated with Syndrome X is a tendency to be low on testosterone. Since testosterone enhances sugar metabolism, fat burn off and circulation, poor lifestyle choices combined with inadequate levels of testosterone can result in Syndrome X.

Stress and Sugar Metabolism

The brain is the first organ to react to elevated sugar or hormones in the blood. Stress of any sort, especially emotional stress, has biochemical consequences. A stressful event will stimulate the adrenal glands to secrete adrenaline, which incites the body's "fight or flight" mechanism. This includes a sudden increase of blood sugar, which stimulates a burst of insulin.

Elevated Cortisol and Adrenaline Due to Stress

As long as the stress continues, the blood sugar remains somewhat elevated, elevating the heart rate and putting the brain on hyper-alert. After a short while, especially if the stress abates, the insulin takes over, blood sugar drops, and the person becomes hypoglycemic. Repeated stressful events result in an increased sensitivity to stress. The person becomes more susceptible to the reactions of stress and to having hypoglycemic episodes even after mild aggravations. This is felt to be one of the possible mechanisms that induce reactive hypoglycemia. As long as the adrenal surge continues, the blood sugar remains somewhat elevated. When the adrenal surge abates, symptoms occur.

Over time, the same stress hormones that function to protect the body may actually upset the sugar metabolism. Cortisol and adrenaline are known as the body's anti-stress hormones because they protect the body during periods of potential danger. When we experience a danger or threat, adrenaline and cortisol are released, causing a rise in blood sugar due to the increased need for glucose by the brain. Rapid heart rate and an increase in blood pressure also prepare the body for fight or flight. Not only do the anti-stress hormones produce hypoglycemic symptoms, but a rise in blood sugar will cause the pancreas to secrete insulin, causing blood sugar to drop. The elevated hormones can linger in the body for days.

Hypoglycemia and Delinquency

Several studies on incarcerated juveniles link hypoglycemia brought on by a diet high in sugar and refined carbohydrates to antisocial behavior. In the early 1980s, Stephen Schoenthaler, Ph.D., studied 276 incarcerated juveniles and found that antisocial behavior was lowered by 50% after sugar was eliminated from their diet. Those arrested for violent crimes showed the greatest improvement.

Attention Deficit and Hyperactivity Disorder (AD/HD)

Learning disabilities such as Attention Deficit Disorder (ADD) and Attention Deficit Hyperactivity Disorder (ADHD) have become widespread in the last twenty years. Researchers report that one out of every five children is diagnosed with a behavior or learning disorder.

In children, the physical, mental, and emotional changes caused by hypoglycemia may manifest themselves as hyperactivity, loss of attention, inability to concentrate, and emotional instability. This can cause a normally pleasant child to have a "meltdown" and act out with temper tantrums.

Many parents discover dramatic improvements by making changes in the breakfast they prepare. Instead of sugary cereals that contain sugar, corn syrup, dextrose, brown sugar, and honey, try high protein/low carbohydrate alternatives. If sweeteners are used, it is best to use either fructose or stevia. Refer to the list later in this chapter for common low glycemic foods to avoid hypoglycemic episodes. You may also refer to diets that have a balanced approach, such as the maintenance stage of the Atkins Diet, The South Beach Diet, or the Zone Diet (See: Resources).

Migraine Headaches

For true migraine sufferers, food does not make a headache disappear. Headaches that are associated with hypoglycemia will disappear shortly after food is ingested.

In a study published in a 1978 issue of the *Journal of the American Medical Association*, researchers Dexter, Roberts and Byer performed tests for hypoglycemia on 74 patients with migraines. Results showed 8% were diabetic and 76% had reactive hypoglycemia. Following dietary therapy that included a low carbohydrate six-meal regimen, 56% of those with reactive hypoglycemia showed a greater than 75% improvement in the frequency and severity of their headaches.

Case Study: Mary

Mary had a problem that she could not put her finger on. She knew that she would get very tired, dragged out, foggy, and almost incoherent, but she could still function—at least to some degree. Her symptoms would come and go throughout the day. She would wake up feeling fine, have breakfast, and then a couple hours later start feeling groggy and a little tired. She usually felt pretty good after lunch. Within a couple of hours, she was tired again and a little irritable. Three hours after a good supper, she would have to have a snack.

Her test results showed that three hours after eating, her blood sugar plummeted. She had reactive hypoglycemia. When she was placed on a balanced high-protein diet, her blood sugar stabilized. In her case, the Zone Diet was most appropriate. Rather than waiting until she was ravenously hungry, Mary was instructed to have a high-protein snack every couple of hours to maintain her blood sugar levels. As her body acclimated to a high protein/low carbohydrate diet, her blood sugar leveled off. Within a few weeks, Mary began losing weight and was thinking and feeling much better. Her hypoglycemia was successfully treated.

Assessing Your Blood Sugar

Although you may need to see your doctor to schedule a test for hypoglycemia, symptoms often provide the best clues.

Questionnaire for Hypoglycemia

The following questionnaire will help you determine if you have hypoglycemia.

Directions

Fill in a value after each question using the following as a guide:

0   = No
1   = Rarely
2   = Sometimes
3   = Always

Question	0	1	2	3
1. Do you crave sweets?				
2. Do you feel irritable if you miss a meal?				
3. Do you have frequent headaches?				
4. Do you feel tired within a few hours after eating?				
5. Do you ever feel shaky?				
6. Do you ever have blurred vision?				
7. Are you depressed?				
8. Do you have mood swings?				
9. Do you get anxious or nervous for no apparent reason?				
10. Do you have trouble concentrating?				
11. Does eating alleviate your symptoms?				

Normally, the glucose level will rise within 1-2 hours and can be as high as 125-130 ug/dl after which it decreases gradually to its original level. If however, the blood glucose levels plummet and the person experiences hypoglycemic symptoms, then the diagnosis is reactive hypoglycemia.

To calculate your score, add the numeric value of your responses. If your total score falls below five, you probably do not have hypoglycemia. If your score falls between 6 and 15, you may have hypoglycemia and if your score is greater than 15, you very likely have hypoglycemia.

Tests for Hypoglycemia

Two tests exist for detecting hypoglycemia. Both involve the measurement of blood glucose levels. Normal fasting blood sugar ranges from 80 to 105 ug/dl blood. When blood sugar drops below 60 ug/dl, there's an adrenaline response to release liver-stored sugar. If fasting blood sugar drops below 60 ug/dl, the diagnosis is fasting hypoglycemia.

Glucose Tolerance Test

An oral glucose tolerance test (GTT) has become a standard test of blood sugar control. After a fast of at least 8 hours, steps for the glucose tolerance test include:

1. A test for a baseline blood glucose measurement
2. A drink containing glucose or a high glycemic index meal
3. Blood sugar levels are measured hourly for five to six hours.

Glucose-Insulin Tolerance Test

Because it is recognized that hypoglycemia can exist in people having blood sugar levels above 60 ug/dl, the glucose-insulin tolerance test measures insulin (or epinephrine or adrenaline) during the test to correlate symptoms with the elevation of these hormones. This test uses a similar five-hour glucose tolerance test combined with measurements of insulin levels. Researchers have found that as many as two thirds of subjects with suspected sugar abnormalities and normal glucose tolerance tests have abnormal insulin tolerance tests.

Dietary Tool: Glycemic Index

Controlling the insulin response is the key to managing both hypoglycemia and diabetes. The glycemic index has become a popular tool for selecting foods that do not put stress on the pancreas. Well-managed insulin levels contribute to the following:

- Increased mental alertness
- Reduced risk of diabetes
- Reduced body fat
- Reduced incidence of high blood pressure

Measuring the Quality of Carbohydrates

Developed as a method for helping diabetics control blood sugar, the Glycemic Index (GI) was first developed by Canadian professor of nutrition David Jenkins in 1981. This tool can also help people who have a hypoglycemic reaction to carbohydrates. The glycemic index has also been useful for athletes who need to manage their blood sugar levels after physical exertion.

Jenkins and his fellow researchers studied how quickly various foods affect blood sugar. His team of researchers assigned a numerical value to foods. The value indicates how rapidly 50 grams of a food will raise blood sugar compared to a food that is known to be rapidly digested (glucose or white bread). The researchers classified foods as follows:

High Glycemic Foods
High glycemic foods (80 and higher) digest rapidly and cause a fast release of glucose into the blood stream.

Low Glycemic Foods
Low glycemic foods (40 and lower) digest slowly and release glucose into the blood gradually.

Previously (in the 1970s), carbohydrates were defined as either simple or complex. Simple carbohydrates such as chocolate and sugary deserts were thought to be absorbed immediately. Complex carbohydrates such as breads, pasta, and potatoes were thought to break down slowly, providing steady, long-term energy.

Jenkins and his team discovered that the categorizing of simple and complex carbohydrates is not accurate. In Jenkin's research, the foods that produced the highest glycemic responses were many of the complex carbohydrates, including white bread, breakfast cereal, and potatoes.

Authors of popular diet books such as *The South Beach Diet, Sugar Busters* and *The Zone* recommend that the GI be used as a tool for managing blood sugar levels. Authors of these books advise readers to counteract the ill effects of high-glycemic foods by combining low-glycemic foods with high-glycemic foods and foods that are high in fiber at the same meal.

Numerous pocket guides containing lists of high and low-glycemic foods are now available to help plan meals. The following chart will give you some basic information about the GI.

Category	Food	Glycemic Index (GI) *High (80-100)* *Medium (40-80)* *Low (1-40)*
Sugars	Glucose	100
	Honey	75
	Fructose	20
Fruits	Peach	28
	Apple	39
	Banana	62
	Orange	40
	Orange juice	46
	Raisin	64

	Cherries	32
	Grapefruit	36
	Grapefruit juice	69
	Pear, fresh	53
	Pear, canned	63
	Plum	55
	Grapes	66
	Kiwi	75
	Mango	80
	Apricots, canned syrup	91
	Pineapple	94
	Watermelon	103
Vegetables	Beets	64
	Carrots (raw)	31
	Carrots (cooked)	36
	Corn, sweet	55
	Potato (baked)	98
	Potato (red skin, boiled)	70
	Potato, yams	71
	Parsnips	131
	Pumpkin	107

Grains/Cereal	Cereal, Bran	51
	Cereal, Muesli	66
	Cereal, Cheerios	83
	Cereal, Cornflakes	80
	Cereal, Rice Krispies	82
	Cereal, Mini Wheats	81
	Cereal, Nutri Grain	94
	Cereal, Oatmeal	49
	Cereal, Rice Puffs	95
	Cereal, Wheat	67
	Bread, Wonderbread	112
	Bread, French Baguette	136
	Bread, Whole Grain	72
	Bread, Pita, Whole Wheat	57
	Bread, Pita, White	82
	Bread, Hamburger Bun	87
	Bread, Kaiser Rolls	104
	Bread, Melba Toast	100
	Bread, Rye	65
	Bread, Mixed Grain	45

	Bread, Pumpernickel	41
	Bread, Sourdough	57
	Bread Stuffing	106
	Rice	70
	Rice, brown	79
	Rice Cakes	110
	Barley, pearled	36
	Wheat, quick cooking	77
	Couscous	93
	Millet	101
	Tapioca, boiled with milk	115
	Cornmeal	98
Pasta	Spaghetti, protein enriched	38
	Fettuccini	46
	Ravioli, meat	56
	Spaghetti, white	59
	Linguini	65
	Tortellini, cheese	71
	Macaroni and cheese	92
	Gnocchi	95

Legumes	Garbanzo beans	47
	Pinto beans	55
	Pinto beans, canned	64
	Soy beans	25
	Black-eyed beans	59
	Kidney beans, canned	69
	Lentils	29
	Peas	39
Soups	Tomato	54
	Lentil soup canned	63
	Black bean	92
Snacks	Peanuts	21
	Peanut M & Ms	46
	Popcorn	79
	Corn chips	105
	Chocolate	70
Other Foods	Ice cream	36
	Milk	34
	Sausage	28

Note: High fiber content in foods will reduce the glycemic index.

Treatment

Effective treatment for reactive hypoglycemia involves stabilization of blood sugar levels with a proper diet. Many of the foods we eat, especially sugar, are capable of upsetting our body chemistry. Depending on the severity of the imbalance, restabilizing the body chemistry may take several months.

People who find that they have hypoglycemia may be totally unaware of how their diet affects their metabolism. Often, a return to a balanced state involves a radical re-education about food.

The severity of your hypoglycemia will determine how much you need to adjust your diet.

Severe Hypoglycemia

If your symptoms include palpitations, dizziness or tremors, a rebalancing of the body chemistry will require that you avoid caffeine and alcohol and eat:

- Low glycemic foods
- Protein at every meal
- Frequent small meals

Besides having a stabilizing effect on the blood sugar, low-glycemic foods will:

- Help eliminate brain fog
- Reduce mood swings
- Reduce fatigue
- Reduce the incidence of type 2 diabetes
- Help control type 1 and type 2 diabetes
- Improve muscle-to-fat ratio
- Not stimulate fat storage

Moderate-to-Light Hypoglycemia

If your symptoms include concentration difficulties, fatigue after eating, or headaches if you miss a meal, a moderate amount of adjustment in your eating habits may be all that's required to control hypoglycemic symptoms. Although low-glycemic foods are preferred, they can be combined with moderate-glycemic foods to slow the release of insulin. Be careful about eating high-glycemic foods and eat them only in combination with low-glycemic foods.

The Consequences of Vegetarianism

Although some people thrive as vegetarians, many people do not understand the consequences of restricting their diet to plant protein. Animal proteins, which include meat, poultry, fish, and eggs contain all 8 essential amino acids and 14 non-essential amino acids required to build important components in the body, such as blood cells, muscle tissue, and antibodies. Vegetarian diets can easily be deficient in essential amino acids. Vegetarians must be careful to combine grains and legumes in order to assemble the appropriate balance of essential amino acids in vegetarian meals.

In addition to the difficulties of assuring an adequate intake of proteins with a vegetarian diet, there is also the issue of the glycemic content of the diet. All too frequently, vegetarians choose diets that may seem healthy on the outside, but contain too many high-glycemic foods, which can be debilitating. So if you are going to pursue a vegetarian diet, you must be certain that your meals are balanced with protein, in addition to balancing the glycemic index.

Artificial Sweeteners

Aspartame

Aspartame, the chemical name for NutraSweet, is one of the most toxic of food additives. Its three components include phenylalanine, aspartic acid, and methanol. Its use in food products is now pervasive, and it is added to products that are sold in over 60 countries. What is particularly insidious is that free methanol is created from aspartame when it is heated above 86° Fahrenheit. Many of the foods that contain aspartame are heated beyond 86 degrees in food processing. Methanol breaks down into formic acid and formaldehyde in the body. Formaldehyde is a deadly neurotoxin.

According to researchers and physicians studying the adverse effects of aspartame, symptoms caused by aspartame include:

- Headaches/migraines
- Dizziness
- Seizures
- Nausea
- Numbness
- Muscle spasms
- Weight gain
- Rashes
- Depression
- Fatigue
- Irritability
- Tachycardia
- Insomnia
- Vision problems
- Hearing loss
- Heart palpitations
- Breathing difficulties
- Anxiety attacks
- Slurred speech
- Loss of taste
- Tinnitus
- Vertigo
- Memory loss
- Joint pain

Stevia

If you need a sweetener, try stevia. Stevia is an herb that is 300 times sweeter than sugar and does not have any reported toxic side effects. Although stevia has never received FDA approval as a food additive, it is sold as a dietary supplement and can be found in most health food stores. It has been found to be stable up to 392 degrees Fahrenheit. Stevia has been approved by the Japanese government for use in food processing and is used in a wide range of foods: pickled vegetables, dried seafood, soy sauce, miso, beverages, candy, gums, baked goods, cereals, yogurt, and ice cream.

Supplements

Hypoglycemia can be controlled in ways other than just diet alone. Although some people do need dietary changes, not everyone will benefit from just a dietary change. Dietary changes may also be difficult due to a person's lifestyle or personal situation. Supplements that can help to control hypoglycemic symptoms include:

B6

B6 can help control one's metabolism, making the body more efficient and stabilizing brain function. Taking a dose of 50 to 300 mg. in divided doses each day can be helpful in controlling hypoglycemia.

B5

B5 is also known as Dexpanthenol or Pantothenic Acid. 100 to 500 mg. a day can control hypoglycemic symptoms.

5-HTP

In some people, 5-HTP can regulate a state of anxiety, making the reaction to hypoglycemia less severe. 5-HTP is also useful in people who have a hard time staying asleep at night. They can fall asleep, but wake up after a few hours and have a hard time falling back to sleep. The typical dose is 50 to 200 mg. once or twice a day, especially at bedtime. When you have taken enough of the 5-HTP and your body is appropriately saturated and fortified, you may experience nightmares or very strange dreams. If this occurs, discontinue use.

Glycine

A low dose of Glycine, an amino acid, is not only sweet but can decrease cravings for sugar. The typical safe dose is 500-1000 mg. 1-3 times a day.

Chromium

Chromium can make blood sugar metabolism more efficient and decrease the fluctuation that can result in hypoglycemia. A recommended dose is 200 to 1000 mcgs. a day.

Vitamin B12

Vitamin B12 given by injection or by sublingual tablets can increase energy levels and decrease cravings, as well as ease fluctuations that result in hypoglycemia.

Caffeine

For some people, oddly enough, caffeine can decrease cravings and fluctuations in blood sugar. For a source of caffeine, green tea is best because it is the most gentle on the system. For some people, green tea eases cravings for food and helps control hypoglycemic episodes. Green tea also has antioxidant properties.

Magnesium Citrate

Magnesium Citrate in two 200 to 500 mg. doses a day has been shown to be helpful, since many hypoglycemics tend to be low on magnesium.

St. John's Wort

St. John's Wort in 900 to 1000 mg. in single or divided dosages may ease anxiety that may result in hypoglycemic episodes.

Note: People who exercise are not only healthier, but they also look and feel better. Exercise seems to control fluctuations of blood sugar. A well-conditioned body uses its caloric intake more efficiently and is less prone to both hypoglycemia and hyperglycemia (diabetes).

Resources

Books

Several published books are helpful for people coping with hypoglycemia.

Excitotoxins: The Taste That Kills
by Russell L. Blaylock
Publisher: Health Press
Neurosurgeon Blaylock introduces the reader to excitotoxins—substances added to food and beverages that damage nerve cells in the brain, and are particularly dangerous to the elderly, children, and those at high risk of neurodegenerative diseases. Excitotoxins include glutamate (MSG) and aspartate (NutraSweet).

Dr. Atkins' New Diet Revolution
By Robert C. Atkins, M.D.
Publisher: Avon Books
Dr. Atkins advocates a diet that is high in protein and very low in carbohydrates, which limits the body's production of insulin. Limited insulin production results in diminished food cravings and a reduction in fat storage in body tissues.

The New Sugar Busters!
By H. Leighton Steward

Sugar Busters! For Kids
By H. Leighton Steward
Publisher: Ballantine Books
Although the central theme in the Sugar Busters! books is weight management, both texts include chapters on the glycemic index as well as glycemic index tables.

The South Beach Diet
By Arthur Agatston, M.D.
Publisher: Rodale Press
Agatston's modified carbohydrate plan includes plenty of high-fiber foods, lean proteins, and healthy fats, while cutting bread, rice, pastas, and fruits.

Lick the Sugar Habit
By Nancy Appleton, PhD.
Publisher: Avery Publishing Group
Nancy's book contains exceptionally well-researched information on the biochemical effects of sugar on the body's metabolism. The updated edition of her book, published in 1995, informs us that Americans consume an average of 149 pounds of sugar per year.

Nancy's presentation on mineral relationships includes the work of Dr. Melvin Page, a dentist who discovered the disastrous effect sugar has on the calcium-phosphorus ratio. As mentioned in Nancy's book, as little as two teaspoons of sugar can cause the body's micronutrient ratios to change radically, throwing the body out of balance. For anyone suffering from severe hypoglycemia, Nancy has created valuable self-help sections that describe foods best tolerated by those with unbalanced body chemistry.

The Zone
By Barry Sears, Ph.D.
Publisher: ReganBooks
Dr. Sears revolutionized high-protein diets with his excellent explanation of the effect that diet has on everything from blood sugar, to diabetes, to inflammatory processes, to arthritis, to heart disease, etc. There are numerous books on how to apply the Zone Diet and to plan meals. If this diet is right for you, the results could be quite dramatic within a relatively short period of time.

CHAPTER 7

Food Allergy

Food-related allergies have symptoms that come and go without a seasonal pattern. Approximately 20 percent of the population has food allergies and experiences year round symptoms of brain fog, fatigue, achiness, stuffy nose, sore throat, rashes, eczema and poor attention span.

Allergy vs. Intolerance

Food allergy is a complex subject and, as a result, there is a great deal of confusion surrounding the terms food allergy, food intolerance, and food sensitivity.

Clarification of Terms

Most doctors, environmental ecologists, and scientists agree on the following terms:

Allergy
Food allergies occur when the body's immune system mistakes a food as harmful and creates antibodies to fight it. This reaction involves the body's entire immune system which begins a battle against the "invading" food.

Classic Allergy
Metabolic or physiological pathways involved in "classic" allergic responses are quite well understood by modern medicine. For example, typical allergic responses involve the presence of allergic "markers" like the antibody IgE *(Immunoglobulin E)* and the release of inflammatory chemicals such as histamine. Symptoms that arise from inflammatory chemicals are clearly visible and often occur within minutes after exposure to an offending substance. Examples include:

- Allergic Rhinitis (hay fever)
- Anaphylaxis (anaphylactic shock)
- Reactive Airway Disease (asthma)
- Atopic Dermatitis (eczema)
- Urticaria (hives)
- Allergic Contact Dermatitis

Although the body's immune system can react to almost any food, it is thought that the following foods account for almost 90% of all food-related allergic reactions:

- Grains (wheat, rye, oats, spelt, and barley)
- Soy
- Milk
- Eggs
- Fish
- Shellfish
- Peanuts
- Tree nuts such as walnuts and cashews
- Citrus
- Sugar
- Corn

Intolerance

Food intolerance is very different than a food allergy, mostly because there is no immune response. Although allergic "markers" such as the antibody IgE are clearly absent in this type of reaction, there are many physiological reactions such as bloating, gas, diarrhea, belching, headaches, lack of mental clarity, and fatigue.

The chemicals in food seem to provoke symptoms that are cerebral in nature, such as: depression, mood swings, extreme fatigue, "fuzzy" thinking, or an inability to concentrate. Not surprisingly, chemical sensitivities are often misdiagnosed as psychological problems.

Common Symptoms of Food Intolerance

Food sensitivities are often misdiagnosed because identification of reactions can be difficult. Reactions can sometimes be delayed 48 hours or more and there are no conclusive laboratory tests.

Identifying Food Intolerance

The best way to identify provoking foods is through careful screening with an elimination diet. If you have any of the following symptoms, you should consider creating your own self-test (See: *Food Elimination Diet*).

Category	Symptom
Cognitive This group is closely related to what might be considered "brain fog."	• Confusion • Attention deficit disorder • Learning disabilities • Mental lethargy • Inability to concentrate
Head and Neck Symptoms Several of the symptoms in this group cause the mental fuzziness associated with brain fog.	• Chronic ear infections • Stuffy nose • Recurrent sinus infections • Earaches • Fluid in middle ear • Hearing loss • Migraine headaches • Dizziness • Runny nose • Tinnutis (ringing or buzzing in the ears) • Itching eyes and ears • Postnasal drip • Sore throat
Psychological Symptoms The psychological symptoms in this group are leading causes of brain fog.	• Anxiety • Depression • Irritability • Panic attacks • Mood swings

Behavioral Symptoms	
Hyperactivity and restlessness are frequently seen in children.	• Hyperactivity • Aggressive behaviors • Angry outbursts • Restlessness
Gastrointestinal Symptoms Gastrointestinal symptoms are thought to arise due to a deficiency in certain enzymes required for digestion of the offending food.	• Bloating after meals • Abdominal pain or cramps • Nausea • Diarrhea • Irritable bowel syndrome • Ulcerative colitis • Crohn's disease • Belching • Candidiasis • Undigested food in stools • Constipation
Respiratory Symptoms The same respiratory symptoms associated with classic food allergies are considered to be the result of a food intolerance if there is no classic immune system response.	• Chronic coughing • Chest congestion • Asthma
Skin Problems Skin problems also fall into the two categories of classic food allergies and food intolerance depending on the presence of IgE antibodies.	• Eczema • Psoriasis • Hives • Dry skin • Fungal infections (toes, fingernails)

Other Common Symptoms This group of symptoms falls outside all of the other categories but may be considered the result of a food intolerance if a problematic food is isolated through careful screening with an elimination diet.	• Sleep disorders • Chronic fatigue • Food cravings • Rheumatoid arthritis • Muscle aches

Lactose and Gluten Intolerance

Lactose and gluten are examples of food intolerances and not necessarily related to allergy. Both lactose and gluten intolerance result in abdominal pain, cramping, gas, diarrhea, and in the case of gluten intolerance, sometimes constipation. Symptoms usually occur within a few hours of eating the offending food substance and can last for up to two or three days.

Lactose
Lactose is the sugar contained in milk. It requires a specific enzyme called lactase to break the milk sugar into useable absorbable forms.

Identifying Lactose Intolerance
If you experience abdominal pains, diarrhea, gas, or bloating after eating any kind of dairy product, you most likely have lactose intolerance.

Treatment of Lactose Intolerance
The treatment of lactose intolerance involves either:
1. Avoiding dairy products entirely; or
2. Taking Lactase (Lactaid) each time you consume dairy products in any form.

Gluten

Gluten, a protein found in grains, is what makes bagels chewy. The less gluten, the more brittle the baked product. Gluten may taste good and be fun to eat, but someone who suffers from gluten intolerance ends up having abdominal pains, cramps, gas, bloating, achy joints, mood changes, diarrhea or constipation, and brain fog.

Sprue
Sprue, also known as celiac sprue, is a specific condition where the person cannot tolerate any kind of gluten.

When someone has intolerance to gluten, the only choice is to avoid gluten-containing products. Gluten-containing grains are:

- Wheat
- Rye
- Oats
- Barley
- Spelt

Food Elimination Diet

One of the most accurate methods of detecting a food allergy is to eliminate all suspected foods from the diet for a period of a few weeks and then reintroduce foods one-at-a-time.

Oligoantigenic Diet

The oligoantigenic or hypoallergenic diet is a selection of foods that are thought to be well tolerated by most people who have food intolerances. These foods include:

- Turkey
- Lamb
- Sweet potatoes or yams
- Non-glutenous grains (millet, buckwheat, rice, and amaranth)
- Bananas
- Cabbage family vegetables such as cabbage, brussel sprouts or broccoli
- Celery
- Carrots
- Watermelon
- Seaweed
- Green beans

The elimination or oligoantigenic diet excludes "high risk" foods that are common offenders, including milk, wheat, eggs, soy, corn, citrus, nuts, chocolate, and coffee.

Selecting the Foods to Eat

If possible, the foods you eat while you're on the elimination diet should be organic so that you do not ingest pesticides. In addition, a common form of food intolerance is an adverse reaction to products that are added to food to enhance taste, add color, or inhibit the growth of microorganisms. Make sure your food is additive-free when on the diet. Chemicals that cause the largest number of adverse reactions include yellow dye number 5, monosodium glutamate (MSG), and sulfites. People with asthma are the most vulnerable to sulfites.

Examples of Foods That Contain Sulfites

Examples of foods that contain sulfites include: wine, restaurant salads, shellfish, dried fruits and vegetables, canned mushrooms, pickles and sauerkraut, vinegar, preserved cheeses, and other preserved foods, gravies, potato chips, trail mix, beer, vegetable juices, bottled lemon juice, bottled lime juice, tea, condiments, molasses, fresh or frozen shrimp, guacamole, maraschino cherries, and dehydrated, pre-cut, or peeled potatoes. Other chemical names for sulfites include: sulfur dioxide, sodium sulfite, sodium bisulfite, potassium bisulfite, sodium metabisulfite, and potassium metabisulfite.

Procedure

An elimination diet is usually followed for two to six weeks by food *challenges* or *tests* that slowly re-introduce suspicious foods. Steps include the following:

1. After following the elimination diet for two to six weeks, start by introducing a food that you suspect causes the least problems.
2. Introduce the food you would like to test for an entire day. Eat several portions of the food or foods from the food group for two or three days and then wait 48 hours. Record details about your test in a food diary (See: *Keeping a Food Diary*).
3. If you react to the food, eliminate it. If not, then keep it in the diet and after a week add the next food.
4. Continue to test foods one-at-a-time until you find a problem food. One week between tests is adequate.

It may take 48 hours for symptoms to arise after ingesting a food to which one is sensitive and five days for those symptoms to subside. If you discover that a symptom does not disappear, you may need to eat fewer foods in your oligoantigenic diet. Once you have found an allergen that causes symptoms, you may want to retest two months later to confirm your findings. Often, when a food is removed for two to three months, a moderate amount of the food can be reintroduced without inducing symptoms. Sometimes, however, a suspected food may cause a more severe reaction when reintroduced.

Food Families and Cross-Reactivity

As you begin your investigation of food intolerance, you may discover that you are sensitive to foods that fall into the same groups. When using a food elimination diet, eliminate all the foods in one family. The following list contains groups or families of common foods:

Actinidiaceace Family
Kiwi

Banana Family
Bananas

Buckwheat Family
Buckwheat garden sorrel

Cashew Family
Cashew
Mango
Pistachio

Cereal Family
Bamboo shoots
Barley/barley malt
Cane sugar
Chestnut
Corn
Millet
Molasses
Oats
Rice
Rye
Wheat

Citrus Family
Grapefruit
Kumquat
Lemon
Orange

Composite Family
Artichoke/Jerusalem artichoke
Chamomile
Chicory
Dandelion
Endive
Escarole
Lettuce

Crustaceans
Crab
Lobster
Shrimp

Freshwater Fish
Perch
Pike
Smelt
Trout
Whitefish

Fungus Family
Mushrooms
Yeast

Goosefoot Family
Beets
Chard
Spinach

Gourd Family (Melons)
Casaba
Cucumber
Honeydew

Pumpkin
Squash
Watermelon

Heath Family
Blueberry
Cranberry

Laurel Family
Avocado
Bay leaves
Cinnamon

Legumes Family
Alfalfa
Black-eyed peas
Carob Chick peas
Green beans
Green peas
Guar gum
Kidney beans
Lentil
Licorice
Lima beans
Locust bean gum
Peanuts
Pinto bean
Soy bean

Lily Family
Asparagus
Chives
Garlic
Leek
Onions

Mallow Family
Cottonseed oil
Okra

Maple Family
Maple syrup

Mint Family
Basil
Mint
Oregano
Sage
Thyme

Mollusk Family
Abalone
Clam
Oyster

Morning Glory Family
Sweet potatoes
Yam

Mustard Family
Broccoli
Brussel sprouts
Cabbage
Cauliflower
Collards
Horseradish
Kale
Kohlrabi
Mustard greens
Mustard
Radish
Turnips
Watercress

Nightshade Family
Bell peppers
Cayenne
Chili peppers
Eggplant
Paprika

Potato
Tobacco
Tomato

Olive Family
Olives
Olive oil
Palm Family
Coconut
Date

Parsley Family
Carrots
Celeriac
Celery
Coriander
Cumin
Dill
Fennel
Parsley
Parsnips

Plum Family
Almonds
Apricot
Cherry
Nectarine
Peach
Plum

Rose Family
Apples
Blackberry
Boysenberry
Loganberry
Raspberry
Strawberry

Saltwater Fish
Bass
Cod
Herring
Mackerel
Flounder

Stercula Family
Cocoa
Cola bean

Keeping a Food Diary

Keeping a detailed record of everything that you eat is an excellent way to track what foods are causing symptoms. A food diary will provide evidence of the changes that take place and provide you with enough detail to look for patterns. Before you begin to keep a food diary, it is important to understand that there are different types of food sensitivities that are categorized according to the type of reaction that occurs.

Fixed Reaction

Fixed allergic reactions are thought to represent 10 to 15 percent of allergic reactions. This type of reaction is the easiest to track. Each time a person eats a particular food, the reaction is the same and remains the same throughout their life.

Cyclic Reaction

A cyclic reaction develops because a person eats a food too frequently. If the food is removed for an extended period of time, the reaction disappears.

Cumulative Reaction

A reaction can also be cumulative. For example, a person can experience no response from eating a small amount of a food but react if more of the food is eaten within a short period of time. A cumulative reaction can also occur if a person is exposed to multiple allergens all at once. Eating an offending food may be safe in a clean nontoxic environment but eating the same food in a smoke-filled environment or during pollen season may cause an adverse reaction.

Delayed Reaction

Delayed reactions are those that usually occur within 12 to 48 hours after a food is eaten, but the delay can occur up to 72 hours. This type of hidden food allergy is much more difficult to detect.

Variable Reaction

A variable reaction involves different symptoms each time a food is eaten. For example, one day you have sinus pain and the next day a stomach ache. This means that the body's immune system reacts differently each time a food is eaten.

Where to Start

Either enlarge the following chart with a photocopier or use the chart as a guide to create your own. Take your food diary with you because you'll need to write down everything you eat or drink. Fill out the diary immediately whenever you eat and don't rely on your memory.

	What did you eat or drink?	Where were you?	How did you feel?
Day and Date			
Breakfast			
Snack			
Lunch			
Snack			
Dinner			
Snack			

Pulse Test

Immunologist Dr. Arthur Coca discovered that when people eat a food they're allergic to, there is a noticeable increase in their heartbeat. In his book, *The Pulse Test: The Secret of Building Your Basic Health*, Dr. Coca teaches readers how to find the foods they cannot tolerate.

Use Your Food Diary

Your food diary will help you record your pulse tests. You'll be taking your pulse right after you eat a suspected allergen and again at 30 minutes and 60 minutes after you eat the food. Add three additional columns to the food diary described in the previous section and label them Pulse/0, Pulse/30 and Pulse/60. A pulse test will complement your food elimination diet and help provide additional clues about your food sensitivities.

Normal Resting Pulse

Before you begin testing possible allergens, you will need to determine your resting pulse. The best way to do this is to take your pulse before you get out of bed in the morning. Here's how to take your resting pulse:

1. Locate your pulse by placing your fingertips on your wrist a few inches below your palm.
2. Use a watch with a second hand and take your pulse for 30 seconds and multiply it times 2 or for a full minute. A normal resting pulse is between 60 and 80 beats per minute.

Investigating the Foods You Eat

Because there are several factors that can increase your pulse, you will want to repeat your pulse test more than once before you draw any conclusions. Here are the steps:

1. Take your pulse after eating a meal that you suspect is causing your allergy.
2. Do not eat any other food, and take your pulse again at 30 minutes and at 60 minutes after eating the food you are testing. Keep a record of the foods you test.

If your pulse increases more than 10 to 15 beats or goes over 85, there is a strong possibility you are allergic to that food.

Food or Drink	Quantity	Time	Location	Activity	Pulse/ 0	Pulse/ 30	Pulse/ 60	Symptoms
Date								

Nutritional Antidotes

Dr. Donald Lepore, who has been called a "nutritional research pioneer," found that many food intolerances are actually nutrients that cannot be absorbed because of another nutrient deficiency. He discovered that when the body is provided with the specific vitamin, minerals, or amino acid that is necessary for the complete absorption of a particular food, the food intolerance is corrected. He called the nutrient that cannot be absorbed an "antagonist" (or allergen) and the nutrient that solved the problem an "antidote."

Muscle Testing (Also Known As Kinesiology)

Although allergens may be found in a number of ways, Don Lepore used applied kinesiology to identify allergens and nutrient deficiencies in the body. Kinesiology is the art of determining muscle weakness when a person comes in contact with an unfavorable substance.

Kinesiology was first developed by an American chiropractor named George Goodheart, who used it to evaluate muscle function and general body imbalances. Goodheart's system of testing is based on the ancient Chinese concept of energy—or ch'i—that nourishes the organs of the body. Ch'i energy flows through channels that form the basis of acupuncture, a medical practice that is 4,000 years old. Meridians are channels of energy in the body and are fundamental to our well-being. His theory is that an imbalance can be determined by checking the resistance of a specific muscle. This feedback is provided through energy meridians in the body.

In his years in practice, Don Lepore used a variation of applied kinesiology to investigate vitamin and mineral deficiencies. Prior to each test, Don first rubbed the thymus to activate acupuncture points of the body. He then rubbed the mastoid gland behind both ears to relax acupuncture points. The person being tested holds a glass vial of the allergen in one hand while the practitioner presses down on the other arm. If the arm shows weakness and goes down rather than being able to resist the pressure, an allergy to that particular food is indicated.

Antidotes to Common Intolerances

In his book, *The Ultimate Healing System,* Don Lepore compiled a list of herbs that contain antidotes for common allergens.

Food Intolerance	Antidotes	Notes
Yeast This group also includes barley, cherries, millet, potatoes, prunes, raisins, rye, and walnuts.	**Mineral:** Zinc **Vitamins:** B-1 and B-6 **Amino Acid:** Lysine	Zinc is abundant in red clover. Lysine is found in comfrey.
Rice This group also includes cinnamon, blueberries, grapes, strawberries, watermelon, wine, and pumpkin	**Mineral:** Manganese **Amino Acids:** Arginine and Proline **Vitamins:** B-6 and B-12	Many vitamin manufacturers use rice as a base for making multicap vitamins.
Wheat This group also includes feathers, wool, dust, detergent, and pet dander.	**Mineral:** Magnesium **Amino Acid:** Histidine **Vitamin:** F	Vitamin E is often made from wheat germ and may not be absorbed properly. Vitamin F is linoleic acid, an Omega 6 Fatty Acid found in poly-unsaturated fats such as olive oil. Black walnut and kelp are high in magnesium. A lack of sodium and histidine will cause an allergy to wheat.

Fat	**Mineral:** Sulfur **Amino acids:** methionine, cysteine, taurine and glutathione	The amino acids methionine, cysteine, taurine and glutathione are all good sources of sulfur. Herbal sources of sulfur are sarsaparilla, fenugreek, eyebright, dandelion, burdock, and fennel. Other sources of sulfur include eggs, garlic, and onions.
Corn	**Minerals:** Potassium, Magnesium **Vitamins:** essential fatty acids **Amino acid:** Histidine	Pills may be coated with a "zein" coating, which is made from corn. Herbal sources of these nutrients include black walnut, kelp, and bee pollen.
Oatmeal and Sesame	**Mineral:** Iron **Vitamin:** B-12 **Amino acid:** citrilline	Yellow dock is a natural source of iron.
Milk and cheese	**Mineral:** Potassium from bananas, tomatoes, and alfalfa.	**Vitamin D:** Vitamin D is made from skin exposure to sunlight, and is also found in cod liver oil.
Citrus This group includes, oranges, lemons, grapefruit, tomatoes, pineapples, tangerines, and cantaloupe.	**Mineral:** Calcium **Vitamin:** B-5 also known as Pantothenic acid **Amino acid:** serine	Herbal sources of these nutrients include Royal jelly and comfrey.

Peaches, Pears, Peppers, Plums, and Nectarines	**Mineral:** Phosphorus **Vitamin:** Niacinamide/Niacin **Amino acid:** L Glutamine	Smoking can cause an allergy to this group, as nicotine displaces niacin in the body.
Tomatoes (part of the "nightshade" vegetable group that also includes peppers)	**Mineral:** Phosphorus **Vitamin:** Niacinamide/Niacin and Pantothenic Acid **Amino acid:** L Glutamine	Royal jelly contains pantothenic acid and niacinamide.
Greens (e.g., celery, cabbage, cucumbers, lettuce, green beans, and parsley)	**Minerals:** Potassium and sodium	Bee Pollen is a good source of potassium. Alfalfa is a good source of sodium and potassium, containing two parts potassium to one part sodium Perspiration causes a loss of three times more potassium than sodium.

When a person's sodium and potassium are low, they become allergic to everything.

Problems Not Related To Allergy

You may be experiencing symptoms caused by food but not due to food allergies. The symptoms could be related to food selection, dietary style, digestion, enzymes, absorption, or deficiencies.

Choosing the Right Diet

It is important to bear in mind that no one diet is good for everybody, but for everybody there is one right diet. If you have the right diet, you will feel:

- Energetic
- Trim
- Not hungry
- Clear
- Mentally sharp

There are four basic diet categories:

> **High protein/low carbohydrate diet** such as the Zone diet, Atkin's, Schwartzbein, Protein Power, and Yeast Connection

> **High carbohydrate/low fat diet** such as Pritikin Plan, Dean Ornish, Macrobiotic Diet, Vegetarian, and Vegan Diet

> **Balanced diet** such as the Blood Type Diet, Metabolic Typing, the South Beach Diet, and Fit after Forty

> **Typical American diet**—high protein, high carbohydrate, high fat, high sugar, and highly processed foods (I call this the "High Five" Diet) which is obviously the least desirable one

Most people find that deciding which diet is best for them usually takes trial and error. You should follow a diet plan for approximately one month. If you feel great and your mind becomes clear and sharp, then you have found the diet that works for you. If you find that this is not the case, keep on looking.

If you would like more concrete guidance, you might want to try Metabolic Typing. Metabolic typing was begun by Dr. Harold Kristal and William Wolcott. A glucose challenge test and salivary/urine pH determine whether you are a fast or slow oxidizer. Specific foods are then recommended for your specific type, and an optimal diet plan is determined.

All of the health-giving diets agree on certain basic principles. They are:

- Eating in moderation
- Avoiding sugar
- Avoiding white flour

- Avoiding highly processed foods
- Avoiding excessive alcohol
- Getting adequate rest
- Exercise
- Adequate water intake
- Stress management

Often, by just following the nine points mentioned above, your overall health will improve dramatically.

Resources

Books

The following medical practitioners have embraced integrative techniques or the blending of conventional and alternative medicine.

The Pulse Test: The Secret of Building Your Basic Health
Arthur F. Coca, MD
Dr. Arthur Coca shows readers how to find their allergies. His step-by-step instructions demonstrate how to discover a pulse pattern to find out what foods and/or inhalants cause the pulse to work beyond its regular capacity.

The Ultimate Healing System
Donald Lepore, N.D.
The Ultimate Healing System is a guide to biokinesiology and nutrition. Dr. Don Lepore was a nutritional pioneer who used kinesiology in his practice for over ten years.

The Parent's Guide to Food Allergies: Clear and Complete Advice from the Experts on Raising Your Food Allergic Child
Marianne S. Barber
Marianne Barber is the mother of a food-allergic son who understands the daily coping skills that are needed when living with an allergic child.

Food Allergies and Food Intolerance
Jonathan Brostoff, Linda Gamlin
Brostoff, a recognized authority on food allergy and author of numerous research studies, and Gamlin, a biochemist and journalist, clarify the difference between allergy and intolerance, explaining the immunological processes underlying hypersensitivity.

CHAPTER 8

Nutritional and Metabolic Deficiencies

Often, people suffer from illness not because of what they have but because of what they do *not* have. Deficiencies in nutrients, enzymes, and absorptive capabilities are frequent causes of illness and mental decline.

Fatty Acids

Fatty acids, which are commonly called fats, play a major role in our health and well being. The appropriate use of healthy fat stabilizes blood sugar, enhances neurologic function, and is a critical component of our cell structures.

Essential Fatty Acids

There are two basic categories of fat: essential and non-essential. Non-essential fatty acids are fats that the body either does not need or can make on its own. Essential fatty acids, however, must be consumed from outside sources, as they cannot be manufactured by the body. There are two essential fatty acids: Omega 3 fatty acids and Omega 6 fatty acids. Omega indicates the location of the double bond in the fatty acid carbon chain.

What Essential Fatty Acids Do

Omega 3 and Omega 6 essential fatty acids serve different purposes, all of which are necessary and *must* be in balance for optimal health and function.

Omega 3 Fatty Acids	Omega 6 Fatty Acids

• Anti-inflammatory
• Increase kidney function
• Increase hormone production:
  o Thyroid
  o ACTH
  o Insulin
  o Growth Hormone
  o Prolactin
  o Progesterone
• Vasodilator
• Decreases antibody response
  • Relaxes smooth muscle; therefore, it is a bronchodilator
  • The major fatty acid of the brain
	• Pro-inflammatory
	• Decrease kidney function
	• Increase Aldosterone secretion
	• Vasoconstrictor
	• Increase antibody response
	• Tightens smooth muscles; therefore, brochoconstrictor (asthma)

Good Guys and Bad Guys

At first glance, it looks like Omega 3's are "good" and Omega 6's are "bad." This is not true. Both Omega 3 and Omega 6 fatty acids are necessary and float among the bipolar lipid membranes of the cells. Every cellular membrane has a need for both Omega 6 and Omega 3. If through our diet we maintain the ideal ratio of five Omega 6 to one Omega 3, then everything works beautifully. The trouble begins, however, when we approach the ratio of the typical American diet, which is closer to 10 to 15 Omega 6 to one Omega 3.

If Omega 3 is depleted, the cell will incorporate Omega 6 instead. When the cell must take in Omega 6 instead of the Omega 3 that it needs, then the cell becomes more vulnerable to injury by free radicals due to the cascade of the pro-inflammatory mediators from the Omega 6 fatty acids. With this imbalance, is it any wonder that our bodies have distorted responses to our environment and age so quickly?

Omega 6 Fatty Acids Respond to Inflammation

Omega 6 fatty acids protect the body by responding to infection and injury. This inflammatory process is essential in fending off bacterial and viral infections and stimulating the healing process to repair injuries by bringing blood to damaged areas. In response to stress, the inflammatory mechanisms raise the blood pressure and conserve fluid to enhance the fight or flight reaction.

Omega 3 Fatty Acids Decrease Inflammation

Omega 3, on the other hand, protects the cells by keeping the membranes softer and more fluid and less prone to injury by free radicals. Because the Omega 3 fatty acids form the backbone of mediators against inflammation, they protect the cell membranes from the destruction of inflammation. Additionally, Omega 3 fatty acids enhance conductivity of nerves. The nerves require insulation in much the same way that electrical wires do. The stability afforded by Omega 3 fatty acids allows the nerves to conduct impulses more efficiently.

Balancing Omega 3 and Omega 6 Fatty Acids

When Omega 3 and Omega 6 fatty acids are in proper balance, especially at the cellular level, the cell membranes become more stable and are less susceptible to damage and injury from free radicals. The cells live longer and function better. For example, if someone gets an infection but has the appropriate Omega 3/Omega 6 balance (1 to 5), then neighboring cells do not get affected by the inflammatory immune response to the infection. Not only is the immune response less virulent, but free radicals produced as a result of the immune response will be less likely to harm other cells.

Free radicals are byproducts of metabolism and are destructive to all tissues. Free radicals are primarily responsible for the damage caused by inflammation and are also responsible for premature aging. Free radicals can injure cells by "punching holes" in the membranes and disrupting the integrity of the cells as well as oxidizing the cell membranes themselves.

Since the majority of us have an imbalance of too much Omega 6 and too little Omega 3, we need to increase the Omega 3 component of our diets, perhaps even in a ratio of one to one until balance is achieved. Then we can get back to a more normal balance of five Omega 6 to one Omega 3.

Benefits of Omega 3 Fatty Acids

If I could recommend only one supplement, it would have to be Omega 3 fatty acids. The benefits of this one substance are so wide in scope that it is foolish not to supplement your diet. Benefits of supplementing with Omega 3 fatty acids include:

- Improved circulation
- Alleviated angina
- Lowered cholesterol
- Stabilized moods
- Enhanced healing process
- Prevented or treated allergies, colitis, depression, schizophrenia, ADD/HD, arthritis, eczema, cracked skin of the hands and feet, chronic illness, strokes, PMS, multiple sclerosis, chronic fatigue, and fibromyalgia.

Basically, any inflammatory condition where the immune system is compromising your health can be improved by taking Omega 3 fatty acids.

Sources of Omega 3 Fatty Acids

There are basically two sources of Omega 3 fatty acids: plant based and fish-based. Plant-based Omega 3 fatty acids such as flax seed oil and hemp oil are ALA (Alpha Linolenic Acid) and must be metabolized into DHA (Decosohexamoric Acid) and EPA (Eicosopentanoic Acid) to be used by the body.

Fish-based Omega 3 fatty acids come primarily from the fat of cold-water fish and are already in the form of DHA and EPA.

Seaweed and algae are rich in Omega 3 fatty acids (ALA). When consumed by fish, Omega 3 fatty acids are metabolized into DHA and EPA. To avoid toxic exposure and avoid depleting natural resources, most fish sold in stores are farmed fish. Farmed fish are usually fed corn and not a normal algae and seaweed diet.

Farmed fish may have less of a fishy taste, but they are almost entirely devoid of the beneficial Omega 3 fatty acids for which they are so highly sought after. One should, therefore, be careful to purchase fish grown in a natural habitat rather than farmed fish. If that is not possible, then you will need to supplement Omega 3 fatty acids with either flax seed oil or fish oil.

Summary: Sources of Omega 3

- Fish oils—cold water fish, not farm raised
- Nut oils—walnut oil, perilla oil
- Flax seed oil

Summary: Advantages and Disadvantages of Flax Seed Oil and Fish Oils

Flax Seed Oil	Fish Oils
<ul><li>Easy to take (liquid or capsule)</li><li>No bad aftertaste</li><li>Inexpensive</li><li>Must be metabolized by the body into DHA & EPA</li></ul>	<ul><li>Do not need to be metabolized to be used by the body so ideal for people with chronic illnesses</li><li>Difficult to manufacture and stabilize</li><li>Brands are available that have no fishy aftertaste.</li><li>More expensive than Flax Oil.</li></ul>

Sources of Omega 6 Fatty Acids

Omega 6 fatty acids come primarily from plant sources. All plants manufacture both Omega 6 and Omega 3 fatty acids, but some, like corn, have an overabundance of Omega 6 fatty acids. Olives, (and therefore olive oil) have both Omega 6 and Omega 3 fatty acids and flax seed, (hence flax seed oil) has a small amount of Omega 6 fatty acids and a predominance of Omega 3 fatty acids. Plant oils that are the richest source of Omega 6 fatty acids are safflower, corn, borage, evening primrose, and olive. Other sources of Omega 6 fatty acids include beef, dairy foods, and pork.

Summary: Sources of Omega 6
- Corn and corn oil
- Olives and olive oil
- Safflower oil
- Borage oil
- Evening primrose oil
- Beef
- Dairy
- Pork

Animals Need Essential Fatty Acids Too

Since animals cannot manufacture Omega 6 or Omega 3 fatty acids, they will only have as much as they are fed. If they are fed corn, their meat will contain an over-abundance of Omega 6 fatty acids and a deficiency in Omega 3 fatty acids. If they are fed natural grasses, their meat will have a rich supply of both Omega 6 and Omega 3 fatty acids. Corn-fed beef and chicken are lacking the essential nutrients, but their sweeter taste and softer texture make them more desirable to the uneducated consumer. Free-range beef and chicken have a richer taste and a more nutritious composition. This goes for milk and eggs as well. Chickens who are free-range and fed a more natural diet and are not being fed corn tend to have more wholesome eggs, darker yolks, and a much higher content of Omega 3 fatty acids.

Case Studies: Emily and Joshua

Emily, a two-year-old little girl, was always coming down with sinus infections and upper respiratory illnesses every six weeks. In addition, she had an itchy rash on her legs and was frequently irritable. When 2 teaspoons of flax oil were added to her diet daily, she stopped getting sick, the annoying rash cleared up, and she was much less irritable.

Joshua, a seven-year-old boy, was distractible, disruptive, and diagnosed with ADHD. When his diet was supplemented with Omega 3 fatty acids, he calmed down and was able to focus.

Nutrient Deficiencies

Nutritional deficiencies should always be considered as a cause or at least a factor in any chronic or recurring illness.

All vitamins, especially the B vitamins, are integral to the metabolic pathways in the cell. The B vitamins provide factors for the Krebs Cycle (Krebs Cycle is the metabolic pathway that turns food into usable energy) and are essential for normal metabolism. Although the body can compensate for deficiency states, eventually it begins to wear out, compensatory mechanisms begin to fail, and cell deficiency symptoms begin to manifest themselves as disease. Heart disease can result from a deficiency of B12, B6, folic acid, or magnesium. Carpal Tunnel Syndrome (a nerve irritation in the wrists that causes pain, tingling, and numbness in the thumb, index, and middle fingers) can result from a deficiency of B6. Fatigue and lethargy can be due to a deficiency of B12. Osteoporosis can be caused by a deficiency of vitamin D and calcium. Deficiency of vitamin A can make you more susceptible to colds and the flu. Night blindness may be a vitamin E or A deficiency. Arthritic joints can be due to B3 deficiency.

Tests to Check for Deficiencies

Although there are tests to check for vitamin, mineral, and fatty acid deficiencies, evaluating one's diet should be sufficient to determine where the deficits lay. Testing can be expensive, and I have rarely found it to be necessary.

Digestive Enzymes

Enzymes are what the body uses to break down the food that you eat into particles that can be absorbed. For the most part, enzymes come from the saliva, stomach, and pancreas. Enzyme deficiency results in food not being broken down appropriately. When food is not digested properly, it is either absorbed in an intolerable state or not absorbed at all. Either way, the net result in a state of deficiency in the body.

Undigested Food and Allergies

When food is absorbed in an undigested condition, it enters the bloodstream stimulating the body's immune system. The net result will be the same as a food allergy with fatigue, irritability, brain fog, rashes, arthralgias, weakness, etc.

Diagnosing an Enzyme Deficiency

An enzyme deficiency can be detected through stool analysis, which also detects the breakdown of food particles in the stool. With appropriate digestive enzyme supplementation, the symptoms will be resolved within a few weeks.

Stomach Acid

The stomach produces acid to break down fats and protein and also stimulates the pancreas to secrete its enzymes. When stomach acid is suppressed, because of either age or medications, food particles go undigested. At the end of the stomach is a sphincter muscle (a sphincter is a muscle that surrounds an opening in the body) called the pyloris, which is the gateway to the intestines. Its job is to keep undigested food from entering the intestines. Sensors near the pyloris detect when the food is digested and tell the pyloris to open. If the body detects that the food in the stomach is not digested properly, it will not allow the food to pass into the intestinal tract. As you can imagine, this creates an interesting conundrum. Since food cannot pass down and out, when the stomach contracts it can only go up, creating a reflux.

Gastroesophageal Reflux Disease (GERD)

GERD is what happens when the contents of the stomach reflux (back up) into the esophagus. Since the contents of the stomach are irritating to the esophagus, what most doctors want to do is decrease the acid production in the stomach so that the esophagus will not be so irritated by the contents of the stomach. This, of course, only further serves to delay the digestive process of food. Eventually, the food does pass down from the stomach into the intestines even though it has not been digested adequately. Undigested particles can lead to food sensitivities, allergies, deficiency states, bloating, gas, irritable bowel syndrome (IBS), abdominal pain, constipation, and/or diarrhea. Usually the first symptoms are fatigue, mental dullness, and/or irritability.

Treatment of GERD

The irony of GERD is that it is usually not due to too much stomach acid but rather too little. Therefore, the real treatment for GERD, in most cases, is to take more acid.

By taking extra acid with meals, usually in the form of Betaine HCl or two tablespoons of apple cider vinegar in a glass of water, one can reduce symptoms of reflux by enhancing the breakdown of food and encouraging movement of the food from the stomach into the intestines.

If you find that taking additional acid does not help the symptoms of reflux, the reflux is then most probably due to food allergy or food sensitivity.

Common Causes of GERD
The most common causes of GERD include:

- Caffeine
- Sugar
- Alcohol
- Stress
- Chocolate
- Drinking too many liquids with meals

Intrinsic Factor
Intrinsic factor is a substance produced by the stomach that enables the body to absorb vitamin B12. Without vitamin B12, one becomes anemic, fatigued, as well as depressed, and can lose cognitive abilities.

Intrinsic factor is inhibited by medications commonly used to treat GERD, such as the protein pump inhibitors, Aciphex, Nexium, Prevacid, Prilosec, and Protonix. It is also inhibited by histamine II blockers, such as Pepcid, Tagamet, and Zantac. Therefore, if one is taking any of these medications it is imperative to also take B12 shots at least once a month or sublingual B12 tablets daily to maintain the body's supply of that particular nutrient.

Bile Acid Deficiency

Bile is produced by the liver, stored in the gall bladder, and squirted into the intestine upon demand to help absorb fatty acids. Without bile, the body cannot absorb the appropriate fatty acids. Without fatty acid absorption, the body begins to break down and goes into disrepair, becoming fatigued, easily injured, and inflamed, and can develop arthritis and colitis. Another one of the symptoms of inadequate bile acid production is obesity. Since fats in the diet produce satiety and therefore decrease cravings for food, without bile to absorb fats one may not experience satiety and may have increased cravings for food. Furthermore, if one does not have enough fats in the body, the body begins to store calories as fat and manufacture the wrong kinds of fats. Poor fatty acid absorption, therefore, can result in becoming fat. Other signs of inadequate bile acid secretion are diarrhea or loose watery stools, light colored or yellowish stools, and foul-smelling stools.

The following are conditions that can interfere with the adequate secretion of bile:

- Not enough stomach acid to break down the fats to signal the gall bladder to secrete bile
- Gall bladder stones
- No gall bladder

If, for whatever reason, you lack bile and are unable to adequately absorb fats, then you may need to take one of the supplements available in health food stores that contain ox bile or some other surfactant that will permit proper absorption of fats. These supplements are to be taken with each meal, usually at the end of the meal; however, some people do better when they are taken at the beginning of the meal.

Resources

Alliances and Organizations

Alliances and organizations that provide valuable up-to-date information include:

Campaign for Real Milk
The Weston A. Price Foundation
PMB 106-380, 4200 Wisconsin Avenue, NW
Washington, DC 20016
Phone: (202) 333-HEAL
www.realmilk.com
www.westonaprice.org

Mercola.com Newsletter
Free e-mail newsletter covering nutrition, medical, emotional therapy and lifestyle choices to improve and maintain total health
www.mercola.com

Organic Consumers Association
Campaigning for Food Safety, Organic Agriculture, Fair Trade & Sustainability
6101 Cliff Estate Rd.
Little Marais, MN 55614
(218) 226-4164
Organic Bytes E-mail Newsletter
Organic News Tidbits with an Edge
www.organicconsumers.org/organicbytes.htm

Book

The following book includes important details about nutrition that have been covered in this chapter.

Know Your Fats: The Complete Primer for Understanding the Nutrition of Fats, Oils and Cholesterol
Mary G. Enig
Bethesda Press
Paperback, $29.95

CHAPTER 9

Infectious Diseases

Infectious diseases remain a common, insidious cause of brain fog. Infections have also been implicated in serious conditions such as arthritis, Sjogren's Syndrome, colitis, sprue, Alzheimer's, amyotrophic lateral sclerosis (ALS, i.e., Lou Gehrig's Disease), multiple sclerosis (MS), chronic fatigue, and Parkinson's. Keeping one's immune system healthy, avoiding activities that put one at a high risk for exposure, and getting adequate rest and nutrition can oftentimes prevent the ravages of infections.

If an infection is the cause of your brain fog, usually one or more of the following symptoms will be present:

- Exercise makes you feel worse
- Night sweats
- Low-grade fevers associated with pain, especially in the evenings
- The more you do the worse you feel
- Desire to sleep excessively yet you never feel refreshed
- Loss of appetite

Why Do Infections Occur?

Infections occur when organisms such as bacteria, viruses, yeast, parasites, spirochetes, or prions invade the body and overwhelm the immune system. Infections are frequently "self-limiting," which means that within a reasonable amount of time they will be eliminated by the immune system. If the body's self-defense mechanism is too weak or the infectious agent too strong, the infections may become chronic and impact one's overall health.

Infectious Diseases and the Immune Response

There are two parts to an illness. The first is the infection, and the second is the body's response to the infection by the immune system. It is the immune system's response to the infection that makes a person feel sick and not the infection itself. Therefore, as important as it is to treat the infection, it is also important to treat the body's response to the infection.

While the immune system is a wonderful mechanism by which the body protects itself, and without which we could not live, the immune system gone awry can be highly destructive.

In this chapter, we will not only be looking at how to eliminate the infection but also how to enhance immune function while at the same time controlling its deleterious effect on the body.

How Infectious Diseases Affect the Brain

Infections usually affect the brain both directly and indirectly. When an infection attacks the brain directly, it will cause brain cells to malfunction or die by interfering with the cells, disrupting the membranes of the cells, or draining energy from the cells. When an infection affects the brain indirectly, it is through the immune system, creating an inflammatory response.

The Inflammatory Response

Once the immune system is activated, it has an indirect effect on the brain. When the immune system senses a foreign substance in the body, be it bacteria, virus, or allergen, antibodies are activated and stimulate the white blood cells (e.g., lymphocytes, monocytes, phagocytes, t-helper cells, natural killer cells) to surround, neutralize, destroy, and dispose of the offensive agent. This attack on the foreign substance is accompanied by increased blood flow to the area. With increased blood flow, the area gets hot, accumulates fluid, swells, and becomes painful. Because of the accumulation of the byproducts that white blood cells produce to kill an invading organism, there is damage to the surrounding tissue. In addition, if the invading virus or bacteria infects the cell walls, the immune system may think that the cell walls themselves are foreign bodies and then begin to attack the body's own tissues.

That Which Was Designed to Protect Now Harms

Many of the chronic diseases are due to the immune system's overreaction or inappropriate reaction, resulting in a myriad of conditions, such as ALS, Alzheimer's, MS, chronic fatigue, rheumatoid arthritis, lupus, and even cancer.

Modulating the Inflammatory Response

Even though inflammation is a necessary part of the healing process, it often causes injury to the body. The body, however, is not defenseless against its own defense mechanism. It produces cortisol to help control the inflammatory response and quell the sense of illness. This usually works well on a short-term basis. However, with aging and prolonged infections, one's coping mechanism begins to weaken, cortisol levels drop, and the inflammatory response accelerates.

Antibiotics: Friend or Foe?

Antibiotics, which kill bacteria, play an important role in the treatment of infections. Antibiotics, however, are a double-edged sword, and while they may be necessary, they must be used judiciously or other problems can result. Overuse of antibiotics can encourage mutations that create hardier bacteria that are harder to kill. In addition, many antibiotics also wipe out the good bacteria in the GI tract (i.e., gastrointestinal tract, which refers to the entire digestive system from mouth to anus). The good bacteria in the GI tract produce B12, process nutrients, and maintain a balance in the body by keeping the bad bacteria in check. Killing off the good bacteria can lead to an overgrowth of yeast in the body, which can create a host of problems such as leaky gut syndrome (where nutrients enter the blood stream without first being digested), chronic fatigue, mood and mental changes, dermatitis (rashes), chronic illness, arthritis, and heart disease, to name a few. That is why it is critical to take probiotics such as acidophilus, bifidobacteria, and enterococcus for at least two weeks after a course of antibiotics to recolonize the GI tract with good bacteria. An anti-yeast medication may also be necessary to keep the yeast in the gastrointestinal tract in check.

Infections for Which Antibiotics Are Indicated

There are certain infections where it does not pay to avoid the use of antibiotics. The antibiotics are extremely valuable, not only in saving lives but also in improving quality of life.

The Tick-Borne Diseases: Lyme, Bebesia, Ehrlichia, and Bartonella

When Lyme Disease was first identified in Lyme, Connecticut, it was thought to be due only to one organism, *Borrelia burgdorferi*. It was soon discovered that the infections being spread by the deer tick included Bebesia, Ehrlichia, and Bartonella. In addition, these infections can travel together in the same deer tick in the same areas.

Furthermore, contrary to popular belief, Lyme Disease is not confined to the wooded areas of the Northeastern United States. Lyme and its associated tick-borne diseases are common throughout the world and are spread not only by ticks but by mosquitoes, blood, and sexual contact.

Symptoms of the Tick-Borne Diseases
All of the tick-borne diseases tend to have the same or similar symptoms: fever, chills, achiness, joint pains, fatigue, sweating, nausea, and sometimes vomiting. Symptoms may not appear for up to three weeks.

Treatment of Lyme Disease
Of the various tick-borne diseases, Lyme is the most insidious and the most dangerous. If treatment is delayed, the symptoms may subside spontaneously and you may feel better without any treatment. This is very dangerous. At that time, the Lyme bacterium, a deadly spirochete, goes into a latent stage able to reappear after months or years have passed (Note: spirochete refers to the shape of the bacteria and its ability to enter a cell and infect it). At that point, brain damage begins, resulting in significant neurologic consequences, such as confusion, slowness of thought and speech, loss of memory, and poor decision making. Cardiovascular symptoms can also result, including heart failure, shortness of breath, and even death.

Late Stages of Lyme Disease

Once Lyme has entered the later stages; i.e., stage 2 and stage 3, it is no longer an acute infection but rather a chronic infection. The Lyme Spirochete burrows into the cells, making it inaccessible to antibiotics. It will also be on the alert for antibiotics. When it senses an antibiotic, it will form cysts where thousands of the Lyme spirochetes gather together to form a little ball making them resistant to antibiotics. They remain in this cyst formation until antibiotic levels drop. At that point in time, the Lyme spirochetes will burst out of the cyst and begin to reinfect the body once again.

Typically, doctors place patients on chronic high doses of antibiotics either orally or intravenously in an effort to quell the chronic infection. This, however, has a very low rate of success at a very high level of expense. People afflicted with Lyme will tend to feel relatively well but only as long as they are on the antibiotics. Once the antibiotics have been completed, the Lyme Disease will then flare once again, forcing them to go back on antibiotics a second, third, fourth time, etc. Remember, Lyme Disease should be treated aggressively with antibiotics in its early stage to kill the infection. If left untreated and the infection becomes chronic, antibiotics will be palliative, not curative. Should this happen, herbal treatment with TAO-free Uña de Gato will be necessary.

Herbal Treatment of Lyme Disease

Herbal treatment of chronic Lyme appears to be the only effective means of eliminating the Lyme Disease or controlling it. To date, the main herb used is Uña de Gato. Uña de Gato, also known at Cat's Claw, must be processed to remove all of the tetracyclic oxindole alkoloids (TOA). This is because the active form of the Uña de Gato is the pentacyclic oxinol alkoloids (POAs), and the TOAs inhibit the POAs from being effective against Lyme. In most cases, the TOA-free Uña de Gato is effective within three to four weeks, and should be taken for at least 6 months.

The reason that you take the TOA-free Uña de Gato whenever Lyme is suspected is because it can attack the Lyme spirochete in a way that antibiotics cannot. The TOA-free Uña de Gato disrupts the function of the Lyme, thereby killing the spirochete in such a sneaky way that the spirochete does not have a chance to hide. Although antibiotics are crucial to take in the early stages of Lyme Disease, once that stage has passed, the treatment of choice is TOA-free Uña de Gato.

Reminder: If you have been in a wooded area or have been around animals in an area known to have Lyme Disease, Ehrlichiosis, or Bebesiosis and after a few days or weeks develop fever, chills, or joint pains, see your doctor immediately for appropriate antibiotics.

Mycoplasma Pneumonia

Mycoplasma, perhaps the smallest free-floating organism, also has pleomorphic tendencies; i.e., it can change shape and appearance. Mycoplasma typically starts as a bad cold or cough and can sometimes evolve into pneumonia. Left unchecked by the body's immune system, it can spread easily throughout the body, and by incorporating itself deep into the cell membranes, change the cell's configuration. These cell membranes now have foreign proteins in them, and the body's own tissue looks like a foreign substance to the immune system. The body's immune system will launch an attack on those cells that have the foreign proteins within them, and the result can be severe damage and even organ failure caused by the immune system.

Urinary Tract Infections (UTI)

Infections of the bladder and/or prostate especially in the elderly can have profound yet insidious symptoms. In certain individuals, a UTI will cause them to feel tired, lethargic, confused, and even have mood changes (irritable or apathetic). Easily diagnosed in a doctor's office, the appropriate antibiotics give relief within one to three days.

Chlamydia

Chlamydia has three forms. Chlamydia trachomatis is responsible for the chlamydia associated with sexually transmitted diseases. Chlamydia psittici is associated with psitticosis and is spread by pigeons. Chlamydia pneumonae usually results in a bad cough and cold that may develop into bronchitis or pneumonia. Chlamydia pneumonia spreads rapidly throughout the body and left unchecked can invade the body's cells, resulting in a variety of conditions including heart disease, vasculitis, brain fog, Alzheimer's, ALS, and M\multiple sclerosis. Similar to mycoplasma, chlamydia can initiate an immune response where the body begins to attack itself.

Treatment of Chlamydia and Mycoplasma

Fortunately, chlamydia and mycoplasma both tend to respond to the same antibiotics: Erythromycin, Azithromycin, Chlorithomycin, or Doxycycline. Usually within three to seven days of taking these antibiotics, symptoms will subside substantially. By properly enhancing the immune system's functioning (see "What to Do When You Get Sick"), you can recover from these conditions within two to four weeks.

Infections For Which Antibiotics Are Not Indicated

Antibiotics are only effective against bacterial infections. This section will deal with non-bacterial infections and include the list of the treatments which have been helpful in treating those infections.

Herpes Viruses, i.e., Herpes Simplex Viruses (HSV)

The Herpes family has many viruses. The most common ones are Herpes Simplex I, Herpes Simplex II, and Epstein Barr Virus. HSV I has been associated with cold sores, HSV II is associated with venereal disease, and Epstein Barr Virus is associated with infectious mononucleosis or "mono." All three of these viruses become most active when a person's resistance is at its lowest. Stress, fatigue, poor nutrition, and trauma weaken the immune system, exacerbating any one of these viruses. This is why mono is so common in young people, especially those attending college, who often do not get adequate rest or proper nutrition. With a suppressed immune system, coming in contact with a common virus can result in a virulent and chronic infection.

Epstein Barr Virus and Alzheimer's

The Epstein Barr Virus is most troublesome when it occurs in a person who already has a certain genetic predisposition called the apo E-4 allele. People with the apo E-4 allele in their genes who get an Epstein Barr Virus-type infection have a high likelihood of developing Alzheimer's. The incidence in some studies has been as high as 90 percent. The virus resides in nervous tissue and when the immune system is at a low ebb, the virus can overpower the immune system and in susceptible individuals can cause irreversible damage to the brain.

The chance of developing Alzheimer's Disease can be reduced by being proactive in your health and taking some of the measures outlined at the end of this chapter.

Cytomegalovirus (CMV)

CMV is a virus that is related to the herpes family of viruses and causes similar flu-like symptoms and can also result in brain fog. If allowed to progress too far, it can result in Alzheimer's, Parkinson's, multiple sclerosis, and ALS. In addition, CMV has been implicated as a cause of heart disease and strokes.

Yeast Infections (Candida Albicans)

Candida albicans is the most common yeast-type organism that infects the body and has nothing to do with the yeast that is used for baking bread (saccharomyces). Candida infections are usually iatrogenically induced (i.e., caused by medical treatments, such as antibiotics or steroids) and can occur in any body cavity, such as the intestinal tract, genitourinary tract, and sinuses.

Candida is naturally found throughout the body but is not considered a problem as long as it is kept in check by an appropriate balance of the immune system and of the natural bacteria of the body's cavities. However, whenever the immune system is suppressed or normal bacteria of the gastrointestinal tract is altered, as may occur when taking antibiotics such as Penicillin, Amoxicillin, Augmentin, and Cephalosporins (such as Keflex), symptoms may arise.

Symptoms
Candida can cause gastrointestinal symptoms such as cramping or diarrhea, or more vague symptoms such as fatigue, weakness, irritability, rashes, poor concentration, lack of focus, sugar and carbohydrate cravings, desire to sleep excessively, non-restorative sleep, vision disturbances, and depression.

Diagnosis and Treatment of Candida
Candida infections are easily diagnosed through a stool culture and analysis. Once diagnosed, there are several avenues to take in treating the infection:

Medications
Nystatin is the simplest, safest, and least-expensive medication to treat yeast infections. It is not absorbed through the GI tract, so there is no chance of

having a systemic reaction. However, it is only good for infections of the GI tract itself. Furthermore, not all yeast-type infections are sensitive to Nystatin. Nizoral, Diflucan, and Sporanox, however, are systemically acting anti-fungals. They are absorbed from the GI tract into the blood, and penetrate all tissues of the body. If a person has a yeast infection of the sinuses, vagina, skin, or a severe chronic infection of the GI tract, these medications are very useful.

Herbal Preparations
Herbal preparations include Citrus Seed Extract, Berberine, Caprylic Acid, Uva Ursi, Oregano, and Aloe Vera. Garlic extract can be applied topically. Although these are not as potent or effective as anti-fungal medications, they may be all that are needed especially if used preventatively.

Homeopathic Remedies
Homeopathic remedies quell the body's inflammatory response and enable the body to heal itself. A homeopathic physician should always be consulted for guidance, as there can be a number of different remedies that address this issue.

Prevention of Candida Infections
Obviously, prevention of yeast infections is the optimal choice. Since yeast infections almost always begin in the GI tract and commonly follow the use of antibiotics and steroids, one should always take Nystatin or an herbal preparation from the time one begins a course of antibiotics and continue for at least two weeks afterwards. In addition, it is important to take replacement bacteria, called probiotics, that include Acidophilus, Bifidobactrium, Lactobacillus, and Enterococcus whenever you take antibiotics or steroid medications.

Remember—Sugar suppresses the immune system and therefore enhances growth of yeast. Avoiding sugar is a necessary component in order to recover from these infections.

Stealth Viruses

The stealth virus is so named because it can mimic a variety of other organisms and can result in sudden changes in personality, very poor concentration, poor memory, mood swings, and irritability. The stealth viruses are very difficult to diagnose and treat.

Prion Diseases

Prion diseases are a category of infection by a non-organism. A prion is a protein that invades cells and alters the genes to produce more prions. It can have terrible effects on brain tissue, causing significant destruction of the brain. The most well-known prion disease is Mad Cow Disease (also known as Bovine Spongiform Encephalitis). Another form of prion disease is the Creutzfeldt-Jakob Disease. These are very slow-growing infections that can be present for 20, 30, or even 40 years before symptoms of confusion and dementia begin to appear. After symptoms appear, the disease progresses rapidly and usually results in death within one year.

Sinusitis

Sinusitis, an inflammation of the sinus passages often confused with sinus infections, can fester for many years causing brain fog symptoms, breathing difficulty, lack of energy, or lethargy. Chronic sinusitis is almost always caused by allergies, structural imbalances, fungal infections, yeast infections, food sensitivities, or stress. Once the appropriate diagnosis is made and the treatment is begun, chronic sinusitis can subside along with all of the symptoms within one to two weeks.

Parasitic Infections

Parasites are common in all parts of the world and are often associated with brain fog, mood changes, poor concentration, fatigue, anemia, weight loss, and the need to sleep excessively. Any time anyone experiences these symptoms, especially after a bout of diarrhea or after having traveled, when no other causes can be found, a stool analysis with microscopic examination will usually reveal a parasitic infection. Once diagnosed and the parasite identified, treatment is very effective and results are rapid.

Cavitations

Cavitations refer to small abscesses in the jaw either from a root canal or tooth extraction where an invasion of bacteria from the mouth festers and causes a slow-growing infection. These bony infections can persist through a person's life, causing altered immune function, frequent illness, arthritis, mood changes, poor concentration, fatigue, and confusion. These symptoms may come and go often-times with no pain. If the doctor or dentist is not aware of this possibility, it can go undetected. The best way to treat this condition is to have the infected site drained and cleaned out by an oral surgeon who is familiar with this condition.

What To Do When You Get Sick

In a non-life-threatening situation, you should first allow the immune system to try to overcome the infection. With three to five days of rest, extra vitamins, and immunity-enhancing treatments, you should be feeling much better.

Listed below are some things you can do to boost your immune system to help it overcome a non-life-threatening condition.

Important Note: One of the major reasons that people get sick is that they are fatigued and/or stressed. Without rest the body cannot heal. In the vast majority of cases, people who developed chronic fatigue syndrome went back to work before recovering completely from the initial illness.

Rest

Rest, rest, and lots of rest.

Chicken Soup

See Appendix for the world's greatest chicken soup.

Homeopathic Remedies

Homeopathy offers excellent remedies that enhance a body's immune response and quell the inflammatory response to alleviate the symptoms of infections.

Colloidal Silver

Sipping small doses of colloidal silver throughout the day can help kill both viruses and bacteria.

Colostrum

This is the immune-boosting substance in mother's milk. Commercially prepared products are from bovine sources and available in health food stores.

Transfer Factor

Transfer factor is the active ingredient in Colostrum that transfers immunity from mother to child. Take 10 capsules a day for treatment and 3 capsules a day for prevention.

Vitamin C

Vitamin C, especially in the form of mineral ascorbates, can be taken in doses of one to two grams every hour. When the body reaches its tolerance level, you may experience diarrhea. Do not worry—it will subside within several hours. Resume taking vitamin C after the diarrhea subsides, but do not exceed the amount that caused the diarrhea.

Glycyrrhizin

Glycyrrhizin is an extract of licorice. It is one of the most important antivirals that we have. Intravenous infusion of Glycyrrhizin remains the mainstay of treatment for Hepatitis C in many parts of the world (except in the United States, despite studies that demonstrate stability, safety, and efficacy). Taken orally it kills viruses, decreases cell susceptibility to viruses, and inhibits arachidonic acid (the necessary precursor to inflammation). Therefore, it has anti-inflammatory properties. It also has been shown to kill H.pylori (the bacteria that causes stomach ulcers) and Klebsiella Pneumonia (the common cause of pneumonia and gastrointestinal infections). The dose is 150 to 300 mg. orally in divided doses; i.e., 75 to 150 mg. twice a day.

Important Note: Glycyrrhizin may increase blood pressure. If your blood pressure is borderline high or if you are on blood pressure medications, be sure to have your doctor monitor you while taking this potent herbal preparation. However, people with chronic infections generally have low blood pressure so there is usually not a problem. Glycyrrhizin may help stabilize blood pressure. Glycyrrhizin can also cause fluid retention, and one may need to increase potassium intake or even take Spironolactone.

Uña de Gato (Cat's Claw)

Uña de Gato has properties that are antibacterial, antiviral, and antifungal. It is most well known for its use in the treatment of Lyme Disease. It must be the TOA-free form of Uña de Gato. The dose should be increased gradually, beginning with one drop of liquid extract twice a day in water and increased gradually up to five drops twice a day in water. The dose should be increased every three to four days, and if you begin having symptoms such as nausea, headache, abdominal cramps, or increased fatigue, decrease the dose and then gradually increase it according to how much you can tolerate. Not everyone can tolerate the full dose, so do not take more than your body can handle. Typically for Lyme Disease, the symptoms are better in four weeks, but the dose should be continued for a minimum of six months.

Omega 3 Fatty Acids

Omega 3 Fatty Acids are anti-inflammatory, and they stabilize membranes, enhance the immune system, and quell the body's overreaction to infections and the immune response.

Omega 3 Fatty Acids are essential fatty acids, which means that you cannot manufacture them—you must ingest them. They can be taken either as flax seed oil or fish oil. Fish oils contain DHA and EPA, and therefore do not need to be metabolized before they can be utilized by the cells of the body. Recently, fish oils have become available in a good-tasting liquid form, which seems to pose fewer problems for many people than the capsules. The average dose is three to six capsules or ½ to 1 teaspoon of liquid per day. The total amount of Omega 3 fatty acids and fish oils to be consumed is between one and three grams a day.

Monolaurin (Lauric Acid)

Monolaurin (Lauric Acid) is the most active anti-viral and antibacterial component in mother's milk. It binds to the lipid protein envelope of viruses and inactivates the virus. It is not effective against polio, Coxsackie, encephalomyocarditis, rhinovirus, or rotavirus (i.e., the common cold). However, it *is* effective against yeast, fungi, staph, some strep, chlamydia, candida, Giardia, H.pylori, and gonorrhea. Coconut oil is 50 percent Lauric Acid. The dose is six to eight 300-mg. capsules a day or ½ teaspoon of coconut oil. Preventatively, take ¼ teaspoon of coconut oil a day.

Important Note: Do not overuse coconut oil, as it is a saturated fatty acid which is solid at room temperature. It is ideal for cooking, but it is not an essential fatty acid and the amount should be kept to a minimum.

Quercitin

Quercitin is a bioflavanoid. Not only is it a good general anti-viral to cytomegalo virus, Epstein Barr Virus, HIV, polio, and herpes simplex 1 and 2 (because it blocks RNA transcriptase) but it is also effective against many kinds of cancers. It is an anti-inflammatory (similar to ibuprofen), an antihistamine, and it detoxifies the liver by increasing production of glutathione. The dose is two to four grams a day in divided doses; i.e., 1000 to 2000 mg. twice a day. There is no known toxicity to Quercitin.

Aloe Vera

Aloe Vera is best in a concentrated liquid. I have found 150 percent to be most effective. Take two ounces three to four times a day therapeutically and two ounces once a day preventatively. It boosts the immune system and is especially good for gastrointestinal infections.

Oregano Extract

Oregano Extract is a very powerful immune-system-boosting herb that is effective for virus and bacteria alike.

Olive Leaf Extract

Olive Leaf Extract has been found to be a potent immune system stimulator.

Echinacea

Echinacea has been shown to be effective in helping the body kill viruses and bacteria.

Zinc

Zinc is an important component of Super Oxide Dismutase, which the body uses to control the inflammatory response and free radical production by the white blood cells. Take 30 to 50 mg. a day, and be sure to balance it with copper in a

15-to-1 ratio. Therefore, if you are taking 30 mg. of Zinc you should be taking 2 mg. of copper a day.

Selenium

Selenium in combination with Vitamin E and Vitamin C was found to be beneficial as early as the 1940s by the United States Army. It was implemented at that time to help soldiers and animals alike resist infections overseas. The dose is 100 to 200 mcgs. per day.

L-Lysine

L-Lysine in divided doses of 3000 mg. on an empty stomach has been shown to be very effective in treating and preventing herpes virus infections and cold sores.

MGN3

MGN3 enhances natural killer cell activity, which has a very potentizing effect on the immune system. It has been found to be effective not only in chronic infections but also against cancer.

Intravenous Hydrogen Peroxide

Intravenous hydrogen peroxide kills viruses and bacteria and at the same time quells the inflammatory response in the body. The dose is 500 ml of 0.03% hydrogen peroxide infused slowly over 1-1/2 to 3 hours—the slower the better. It cannot be taken with any antioxidants or free radical scavengers such as vitamin C, because they will neutralize its effect. Many state medical boards persecute physicians who perform this kind of therapy, despite its track record of safety and efficacy.

Ozone Therapy

Ozone therapy infuses ozone directly into the bloodstream. It kills viruses and bacteria and enhances recovery from infections, especially chronic infections. Only a few states permit its use, despite its safety.

Hyperthermia

Hyperthermia, bringing the body up to a very high temperature and creating a very high fever for an hour and repeating it weekly for 3 to 10 weeks, can have profound effects on chronic infections. At high temperatures, such as 108°F, bacteria and viruses cannot live. This is a very specialized treatment that should only be done by those who are highly skilled and experienced in this kind of therapy.

Lymphatic drainage

Lymphatic drainage is a technique employed by the early Osteopathic physicians in America that saved the lives of tens of thousands of people during the flu epidemic in the early 1900s. It enhances the body's ability to drain and clear infections and improves circulation. Most Osteopathic physicians who do Osteopathic manipulation will be able to provide this service. Some physical therapists and massage therapists also perform lymphatic drainage therapy.

What To Use And When

Since everything works for somebody and nothing works for everybody, how does one decide which to try first? Most people find that one or two things work best for them. First and foremost, DO NOT TAKE EVERYTHING ALL AT ONCE: it will not work and it will make you sick! If you are not fortunate enough to have a physician or naturopath available who can help guide you through the choices, here are some guidelines:

Chicken soup

Chicken soup is good food, good hydration, good electrolytes, and it wouldn't hurt!

Homeopathy

Homeopathy is always safe and a good first choice to control symptoms. You may want to consult one of many family guides for homeopathy and follow treatment for your symptoms or consult with a homeopath.

Lymphatic drainage techniques

Lymphatic drainage techniques are always beneficial, always feel good, and are generally without side effects. They enhance the body's immune system, enhance the body's ability to clear infections on its own, and it may be all that you need.

Guidelines for Specific Types of Infections

Use the following guidelines for specific types of infections:

Acute sinus infections
If the above suggestions do not help, I would first try oregano extract and/or olive leaf extracts, glycyrrhizin, transfer factor, or colostrum.

Chronic Sinus Infections
For chronic infections, always think allergies and fungal infections of the sinuses.

Coughs, Colds, Bronchitis, Pneumonia
Aloe vera juice, two ounces three to four times a day with colloidal silver and echinacea and/or golden seal extract.

Severe chronic infections that do not respond to antibiotics
First try intravenous hydrogen peroxide, then MGN3, and then hyperthermia.

If you do not respond to any of these treatments, see your physician or naturopath for guidance.

Prevention is of course the best. Take selenium, zinc, vitamin E, and vitamin C on a regular basis, get adequate rest, good hydration, exercise, and a keep to a low- or no-sugar diet.

Steroids

Attacking the offending microorganism, be it a virus or bacteria, is only one aspect of treating the patient. The other is to control the inflammatory response that is set off by the infections.

Steroids refer to a group of hormones whose basic structure is fashioned from a cholesterol molecule. Included in this class of hormones are adreno-corticoid steroids produced by the adrenal gland (e.g., Cortisol and Aldosterone) and gonadal or sex steroids (e.g., testosterone, estrogen, and progesterone) produced by the gonads (testicles, uterus, and ovaries). Cortisol, or hydrocortisone, is a steroid that is anti-inflammatory. The body produces 10 mg. a day of cortisol. Like everything else in the body, there has to be a balance. Without cortisol, the immune system goes out of control and causes tissue breakdown, inflammation, rashes, and all kinds of problems. When a person is under stress, cortisol levels will rise, causing the body to retain sodium, alter cellular metabolism, slow down glucose metabolism, elevate glucose levels (causing weight gain), slow down circulation decreasing blood flow, and inhibit the action of white blood cells and the immune system in general. Initially, cortisol creates a sense of well being, almost euphoria, and a reduction of symptoms. However, with prolonged stress or adrenal insufficiency, cortisol is depleted, leading to chronic fatigue, inability to cope, brain fog, irritability, and increased allergies.

The Use of Steroids

Steroids can suppress symptoms from a variety of illnesses, and give a person a sense of overall well being. The cortico steroids decrease arthritic pain, decrease fever, improve the appetite, decrease the need for sleep, and elevate the mood.

If steroids do all of these wonderful things, why are they so bad? The reason is that the sense of well being and euphoria are only temporary. The inappropriate use of steroids will decrease blood flow, delay the healing process, suppress the immune system causing infections to worsen, and can result in brain damage, memory loss, mood alterations, heart disease, osteoporosis, severe bone damage (such as avascular necrosis of the femoral head—"hip rot," which necessitates hip replacement), weakening tendons and ligaments making them more prone to injury, weight gain, infertility in both men and women, aggression, insomnia, and distorted body shape.

Steroids have their place. I have seen many people's lives saved by the judicious use of steroids. On the other hand, I have also seen people whose lives have been compromised and even ruined by overuse of steroids.

I consider the following inappropriate use of steroids:

- Injections of steroids for bursitis and tendonitis when other nontoxic means such as Prolotherapy are available

- IV steroids for chronic pain conditions
- 20 mg. or more of prednisone for any condition for more than 1 month
- Chronic use of inhaled steroids for asthma, especially in children
- Steroid drops in the eyes for more than four days

There are many ways to control an overactive immune system without the use of steroids. Finding and treating the cause of the problem through use of non-toxic means would be my first course of action.

Since the inflammatory response often involves the body's production of free radicals (destructive, irritating, and toxic substances used by white blood cells that kill bacteria and viruses), anything that will help absorb free radicals or reverse the damage done by free radicals will enhance the body's ability to recover and limit the impact of the inflammation on the body. The following are a few suggestions:

Vitamin C
Vitamin C, especially mineral ascorbates, is the classic free radical scavenger.

Vitamin E
Vitamin E, 400 to 800 units a day, taken with vitamin C for better absorption.

Coenzyme Q10
Coenzyme Q10 helps repair membranes damaged by free radicals and is particularly helpful in repair and maintenance of the mitochondria (the power plant of the cell). Since it is an expensive supplement, I recommend a blood test to see if there is a deficiency of CoQ10. This is important, because if the body does not need it, it will not absorb it no matter how much you take. Before starting to take CoQ10, make sure that you need it.

Alpha Lipoic Acid
Alpha lipoic acid is a very powerful antioxidant that reverses damage caused by free radicals and is especially important for diabetics because of the high level of free-radical production associated with elevated glucose levels. Taking 100 to 200 mg. a day is all that is needed.

NADH
NADH is a powerful antioxidant that is difficult to keep on the shelf, as it breaks down rapidly, but does help repair damage caused by free radicals.

Bromelain
Bromelain is an enzyme extracted from pineapple that inhibits the inflammatory response in the body. Take on an empty stomach.

Astragalus (Frankinsence)
Astragalus is an excellent ayurvedic herb that enhances the immune system as well as quelling the inflammatory response.

Digestive Enzymes
Digestive enzymes decrease inappropriate inflammatory responses in the body. To control inflammation, they must be enteric coated and taken between meals. To enhance digestion, it is best that they come in capsules and be taken with meals.

Prevention

We must not be cavalier about our health. Adequate rest, appropriate diet, good quality multi-vitamins, and regular exercise are key factors in promoting health and well being and preventing illness and injury. Obviously, life is not perfect and things rarely go as planned; nevertheless, we must make an effort to try to maintain our health, because once it is lost it is difficult to regain.

Things one can take to decrease the likelihood of getting sick:

Adequate Rest

You have gotten adequate rest when you wake up spontaneously and feel refreshed. You should not need more than eight hours of sleep a night, and usually not less than 6 hours.

Vitamin A

It is my experience over the past 15 years that one or two oral doses of 400,000 units of Vitamin A is preventative for the flu and colds in general. Patients who have taken Vitamin A but have not received the flu shot have fared better than their peers who opt to take the flu shot and not take Vitamin A. (Vitamin A can be taken in conjunction with the flu shot.)

Important Note: High doses of Vitamin A should not be given to women who are, or might become pregnant within four months, nor to people with a diagnosis of hepatitis, or to those who already have a high Vitamin A intake; e.g., 20,000 units a day or one cup of carrot juice a day.

High Quality Multi-Vitamin

The degree of potency is not the issue, but rather the balance and the quality. If uncertain as to which multi-vitamin to take, consult a physician or health care professional familiar with nutritional supplements.

Extra Vitamin C

500 to 1000 mg. twice a day.

L-Lysine

500 to 1000 mg. twice a day.

Colostrum and/or Transfer Factor

Colostrum and/or Transfer Factor once or twice a day.

Olive Leaf Extract

One capsule a day.

Aloe Vera Juice

150% two ounces a day.

Massage, manipulation, or acupuncture

By keeping the body structurally sound, its function is improved, the immune system is enhanced, and illness can be prevented.

One need not do all of the treatments to enhance one's health. Usually one or two is all that a person needs, and those are discovered by trial and error. Once you find a pattern that works well for you, stick with it, because remember: what works, works.

By keeping one's immune system healthy, avoiding activities that put one at high risk for exposure to infections, getting adequate rest and nutrition and using outside agents, be they herbs, vitamins, or antibiotics if needed, many of the ravages of infections can be prevented.

Resources

Alliances and Organizations

Alliances and organizations that provide valuable up-to-date information include:

The Weston A. Price Foundation
PMB 106-380, 4200 Wisconsin Avenue, NW
Washington, DC 20016
Phone: (202) 333-HEAL
www.westonaprice.org

Life Extension Foundation
1100 W. Commercial Blvd.
Fort Lauderdale, FL 33309
(954) 766-8433 or (800) 544-4440
www.lef.org/

Chapter 10

Toxins

A toxin is anything that pollutes and poisons the body. Brain fog resulting from toxic build-up can range from occasional forgetfulness and short-term memory loss all the way to profound Alzheimer's dementia. When toxins cause brain fog, loss of brain function occurs slowly. People may simply attribute it to aging or stress. However, as brain function begins to decline over the years, it becomes quite noticeable to everyone.

Besides brain fog, other signs of possible toxic build-up include acne, dark circles around the eyes, headaches that are sometimes accompanied by indigestion, arthritis, premature aging, mood changes, chronic fatigue, depression, and heart failure. In this chapter, we will discuss three common toxins: metals, chemicals, and radiation.

Toxic Metals

Metals that serve no nutritional purpose, such as mercury, arsenic, lead, aluminum, and cadmium, are toxic even in minute amounts. Other metals that are necessary nutrients, such as copper, iron, zinc, and potassium, become toxic at higher dosages or when they are out of balance with other nutrients in the body. Not only do toxic metals harm our cells, but invading microorganisms often thrive in a heavy-metal environment. Researchers in both the U.S. and Europe have shown that microorganisms accumulate in areas of the body that are polluted with toxic metals. Toxic metals can impair mental and neurological functions and alter numerous metabolic processes, causing problems in energy production, the nervous system, the cardiovascular system, the body's detoxification pathways, and the gastrointestinal tract, as well as the endocrine and reproductive systems.

Toxic waste dumps, air pollution, chemical products, mercury fillings, lead paint, tap water, and chemical residue in food have dramatically increased our exposure to metals in the past 50 years. Personal care products such as cosmetics, antiperspirants, mouthwash, soap, shampoo and other hair care products are also common sources of exposure to metals.

Mercury and Brain Function

Mercury is a metal that has an insidious effect on brain function. It is one of the most toxic substances in our environment, perhaps second only to arsenic. Mercury is a metal that, at room temperature, is both liquid and gas. Mercury is used in the processing of chemicals and is found in abundant quantities in fossil fuels, especially coal. When coal is burned, the mercury vapors escape into the atmosphere and are estimated to exceed hundreds of millions of tons a year. Mercury is used in the textile industry. It is used in vaccines (e.g., thimerosal) to totally inactivate any virus that might be harbored within the vaccine. (Fortunately there is a movement now to remove all mercury from the vaccine industry.) Mercury is used in herbicides and as a fungicide to protect seeds from going bad.

Through its use and processing by the industrialized world, mercury enters our environment. Fallout from manufacturing agribusiness and using fossil fuel for energy has rendered all waterways around major metropolitan areas mercury toxic.

Among the vast list of symptoms attributed to mercury toxicity, the most common are chronic fatigue, joint pain and depression. Mercury has a propensity for nervous tissue and can have a serious effect on brain and nerve function. It is present in the environment in two forms: inorganic and organic.

Inorganic (Elemental) Mercury

Inorganic mercury comes primarily from silver dental amalgams. Silver dental amalgams are approximately 50 percent mercury. The level of mercury found in the brain is directly proportional to the amount of fillings in the teeth. In a study of 101 people, 50 of which did not have silver fillings, the following observations were made:

- Those who had more fillings reported more emotional disturbances, anxiety, suicidal tendencies, nightmares, poor concentration, lack of confidence, difficulty in making decisions, and poor attention span.
- After removal of the fillings and subsequent mercury detoxification, participants reported increased tolerance of stress, decreased incidence of depression, improved memory, improved self-confidence, decreased cravings for sweets, a decrease in fatigue, increased stamina, and an overall improved sense of well being.

Entry into the Brain

Although inorganic mercury is poorly absorbed from the intestinal tract, it is well absorbed from the lungs and mucosa of the mouth and nose. Inorganic mercury enters the brain in one of three ways:

- Vapors can be inhaled and absorbed through the lungs, where it passes into circulation, crossing the blood brain barrier. It is taken up by the brain and retained there.
- As it is released from fillings, it is passed directly through the roof of the mouth to the brain via the sinuses. As a result, it is more toxic than mercury that is absorbed through the lungs.
- It can be converted by the bacteria in the mouth and the gastrointestinal tract into organic mercury, which is then readily absorbed through the intestines.

Impact on Reflexes

In addition to affecting the brain, inorganic mercury also has a propensity for nervous tissue outside of the brain and can slow reflexes, making one more prone to injury.

Organic Mercury

Organic mercury comes primarily from consuming fish or other seafood products, or by metabolizing inorganic mercury that leaches from dental silver fillings. It is readily absorbed from the gastrointestinal tract and binds to the red blood cells. It can cross the blood brain barrier, as well as the placental barrier. Because mercury so easily crosses the placenta, it can become concentrated in the unborn fetus. High levels of mercury have been associated with mental retardation in children.

Organic Mercury and the Liver

Organic mercury accumulates in the liver. Since the liver is the primary organ for detoxification of the body, it filters out heavy metals and tries to process them out through the feces. However, beyond a certain threshold, the liver is unable to cope with high levels of mercury exposure and begins to become a "toxic waste site." Normally, the liver produces glutathione (which is the body's most potent antioxidant) to detoxify itself and protect it and the rest of the body from harm. Mercury, however, consumes glutathione and diminishes the liver's ability to detoxify itself. A toxic liver usually means a propensity for developing illness, weakness, allergies, and fatigue, as well as making the person more susceptible to adverse affects from medications.

Glutathione Production and Mercury

Toxins in the body generally increase production of free radicals. The destructive effects of free radicals are eliminated by antioxidants. The major antioxidant in the brain is glutathione. Hence, low levels of glutathione can have a damaging effect on the brain due to the increase in free radicals. A vicious cycle begins. The better the liver does its job to filter out mercury and other heavy metals in the body, the more the mercury accumulates in the liver and the more glutathione is used up, which makes the liver more toxic. Since glutathione is necessary to process mercury out of the body, as glutathione production decreases, mercury accumulation increases and the liver gets even sicker. This is a true "Catch 22." The better the liver does its job, the sicker it gets. (We will learn how to revitalize the liver later on in this chapter.)

Organic Mercury and the Food Chain

Organic mercury begins as inorganic (or elemental) mercury. It enters the food chain through the waterways by one of two means. As rain falls through mercury-polluted air, it picks up the mercury and then dumps it either directly or indirectly into the waterways and/or oceans. The second way mercury enters the waterways is simply from industrial pollution. In either case, inorganic mercury enters the water, and the algae and seaweed absorb the mercury and convert it to organic mercury. The organic mercury is incorporated into the plant, which is then consumed by fish. Little fish that eat the algae and seaweed are then consumed by bigger fish, which in turn are consumed by bigger fish, all the while accumulating more and more mercury. When we eat the fish, we then absorb the mercury that the fish contains.

The Irony of Fish

Since mercury is toxic to all living beings, in order for fish and algae to survive in a mercury-polluted environment, they had to adapt. The adaptive process involves combining the mercury with selenium, creating mercury selenite, which in effect neutralizes the mercury. Combined with Omega 3 fatty acids produced by the algae, and then converted into docosahexaenoic acid (DHA) and eicosapentaenoic acid (EPA) by the fish, the mercury from fish may not be as toxic as was once thought.

Farmed Fish

In an effort to avoid contaminated fish, fish farms were developed to produce fish in a toxin-free environment. Although the fish grown on farms are devoid of mercury and other pollutants, they are also devoid of the benefits of seaweed and algae. It is the seaweed and algae that gives the fish the Omega 3 fatty acid building blocks necessary to produce the desired DHA and EPA. Since farmed fish are fed corn and other substances that lack Omega 3 fatty acids, the fish meat also lacks Omega 3 fatty acids. Therefore, although the farmed fish may be void of toxins, at the same time they are devoid of the beneficial Omega 3 fatty acids.

If You Eat Fish Get Checked for Mercury

The jury is still out on whether or not the mercury in cold-water fish such as tuna, halibut, and salmon is toxic or not. For that reason, if you do enjoy eating cold-water fish frequently, you may want to check your mercury levels once a year.

Lead and Cadmium

According to the U.S. Centers for Disease Control (CDC), lead poisoning can cause learning disabilities, behavioral problems, and at high levels, seizures, coma, and even death. Lead is also linked to higher rates of crime, attention deficit disorder, hyperactivity, and learning disabilities, as well as heart disease, kidney disease, and dental caries.

Lead Poisoning In Children

An April 2003 article in the *New England Journal of Medicine,* demonstrated that even very low levels of lead can affect a child's IQ by as much as 10 percent.

Until the early 1970s, lead was used as an ingredient in U.S. gasoline and paint. As a result, homes built prior to the 1970s may contain leaded paint that can be ingested by children in the form of paint chips or flakes. Lead poisoning is particularly harmful to children. According to Dr. Marc Lappe, director of the Center for Toxins and Ethics, "Lead has been proven to produce insidious damage to health because it threatens the normal development of mental faculties and social behavior, especially in children."

Silicofluorides and the Cellular Uptake of Lead

Fluoride, the chemical used to fluoridate drinking water, is associated with an increase in blood lead levels. This is particularly true when silicofluorides are used for water treatment. Silicofluorides are cheaper than sodium fluoride, the chemical most known for studies associated with the prevention of tooth decay. Many communities opt to use the cheaper chemical, thinking that silicofluoride comes apart, freeing the fluoride for incorporation into tooth enamel. Unfortunately, silicofluorides do not separate completely and this chemical increases the cellular uptake of lead and aluminum. Research recently published in the *International Journal of Environmental Studies* showed that blood lead levels are higher in children living in communities where the water is treated with silicofluorides.

Fluoride

There is mounting pressure in communities all over the world to ban water fluoridation because of its toxic effects on human health. Fluoridating water forces people to drink a chemical that may depress the thyroid and contribute to increased cholesterol, heart disease, depression, fatigue, and weight gain, as well as muscle and joint pain.

The Case against Fluoride

In 1981, Dean Burk, Chief Chemist at the National Cancer Institute, testified at congressional hearings that over 10,000 cancer deaths each year are attributable to fluoridation. His data has been verified by international research, as well as by other congressional hearings.

Since 1990, The National Cancer Institute and the Safe Water Foundation have found the incidence of osteosarcoma, a type of bone cancer, to be far higher in young men exposed to fluoridated water as compared to those who were not.

In the March 1990 issue of the *New England Journal of Medicine,* Mayo Clinic researchers found that fluoridation increased hip fracture rate and bone fragility.

Reasons to Oppose Fluoridation

On March 6, 2002, Dr. Paul Connett, Professor of Chemistry at St. Lawrence University in New York, published *50 Reasons to Oppose Fluoridation.* Here are some highlights:

1. Fluoride is a cumulative poison. Only 50% of the fluoride we ingest is excreted through the kidneys. The remainder accumulates in our bones, pineal gland, and other tissues.
2. Fluoride is very biologically active even at low concentrations. It interferes with hydrogen bonding, which is central to the structure and function of proteins and nucleic acids.
3. A recent study in the U.S. found increased rates of infertility among women living in areas with 3 or more parts per million (ppm) of fluoride in the water. According to this study published in the *Journal of Toxicology and Environmental Health,* "Most regions showed an association of decreasing total fertility rate (TFR) with increasing fluoride levels."
4. Early symptoms of skeletal fluorosis, a fluoride-induced bone and joint disease that impacts millions of people in India, China and Africa, mimic symptoms of arthritis. Few if any studies have been done to determine if the high prevalence of arthritis in America (over 42 million Americans) is related to our growing fluoride exposure.
5. Other sources of fluoride include food processed with fluoridated water, fluoridated dental products and, pesticide residues on food.
6. The chemicals used to fluoridate water in the U.S. are not pharmaceutical grade. Instead, they come from the wet scrubbing of the superphosphate fer-

tilizer industry. These chemicals (90% of which are sodium fluorosilicate and fluorosilicic acid), are classified as hazardous wastes contaminated with toxic metals and trace amounts of radioactive isotopes. Recent testing by the National Sanitation Foundation suggests that the levels of arsenic in these chemicals are high and of significant concern.

7. Some of the earliest opponents of fluoridation were biochemists. At least 14 Nobel Prize winners are among the scientists who have expressed their reservations about the practice of fluoridation.

8. The 2000 recipient of the Nobel Prize for Medicine and Physiology, Dr. Arvid Carlsson of Sweden, was one of the leading opponents of fluoridation in Sweden. He was part of the panel that recommended that the Swedish government reject the practice, which it did in 1971.

Lead and Cadmium in Chocolate

In May, 2002, the American Environmental Safety Institute sued chocolate manufacturers in Los Angeles County Court, saying that research shows that dangerous levels of lead and cadmium in chocolate pose a serious health risk, especially to children. The environmental group cited chocolate manufacturers for violating California's Proposition 65, a consumer health law that requires warnings to be given to individuals before they are exposed to hazardous and dangerous chemicals.

Aluminum

Aluminum is a ubiquitous element in the earth's crust that is also found in air and water. Because of its light weight and resistance to rusting, it is used extensively in industry for commercial as well as private use.

Aluminum and Free Radicals

Aluminum incorporated within the body can be a major source of free radicals. Free radicals are capable of wreaking havoc on tissue because they oxidize membranes, break down tissue, and poke holes in cell walls and membranes, thus disrupting their function. This destructive process, of course, leads to degeneration of joints, the brain, the heart, and vascular tissue, causing pain and loss of function. The effect of aluminum accumulation on the brain is a loss of memory, loss of mental abilities and faculties, mental confusion, depression, and mood changes.

Aluminum and Alzheimer's

Aluminum is frequently found in the brains of victims of Alzheimer's Disease. We do not know if the accumulation of aluminum in the brain is responsible for the progression of Alzheimer's dementia or if it is a pathologic process associated with Alzheimer.

Whether aluminum is a cause or effect of Alzheimer's, the bottom line is that aluminum is bad. As such, exposure and consumption of aluminum must be kept to a minimum.

Sources of Aluminum

Aluminum is a popular metal used to make pots and pans and, of course, aluminum foil. Cooking with aluminum cookware, especially with acidic foods, causes aluminum to leach into the foods. Other sources of aluminum are antacids, buffered aspirin, antiperspirants, bleached flour, cream of tartar, Parmesan cheese, processed cheese, and even pickles. You must be careful to read the labels before you utilize any of these products in order to avoid taking in aluminum.

Studies have shown that in the presence of fluoride, aluminum leaches out of cookware. Boiling fluoridated tap water in an aluminum pan leaches almost 200 parts per million (ppm) of aluminum into the water in 10 minutes.

Arsenic

Arsenic causes the same problems that mercury does in the brain and body and may be even more toxic then mercury.

Sources of Arsenic

- Fish from contaminated waterways and industrialized areas

- Pressure-treated wood contains arsenic that leaches out and should never be used in the home, a closed environment, on eating surfaces, or where children are playing.

Testing and Treatment for Arsenic

Testing and treatment for arsenic toxicity is the same as for mercury toxicity.

Diagnosing Metal Toxicity

The easiest way to diagnose metal toxicity is via the Dimercaptosuccinic acid (DMSA) Challenge Test. There are several labs that reliably test urine for heavy metals. Two of the most popular ones are Doctor's Data and Great Smokies. They offer panels that check for all of the toxic metals. The DMSA Challenge Test is based on the fact that DMSA is capable of binding toxic metals and causing them to be excreted from the body into the urine. Without the DMSA, the metals may not appear in the urine at all. To take the DMSA Challenge Test you must:

- Empty the bladder.
- Take 500 mg. of DMSA.
- Collect all urine for 12 hours (easiest when done overnight).
- Send in a sample of the urine to the lab.

Urine Analysis for Heavy Metals

I prefer urine analysis over hair analysis when testing for heavy metals, for the following reasons:

- **There is inconsistency** among labs that test the hair for heavy metals.
- **Hair analysis can be very confusing.** For example, high levels of mercury in the hair can mean that the body is excreting mercury effectively and therefore there is little accumulation in the body, or it can mean that the body does have high levels of toxins. Low levels of mercury in the hair can mean that the body either has low levels of mercury, or the body is unable to excrete it in the hair, therefore indicating high levels in the body.

Removing Toxins: Self-Help Measures

Many self-help measures that remove metals also remove other toxins, as well.

Decrease Exposure

Reduce exposure to metals by filtering your water, and by replacing aluminum cookware with stainless steel, clay, or glass cookware. Avoid living in toxic environments where pollution is heavy.

Hydration

Being well hydrated allows the body to excrete toxins through the kidneys. Water consumption should be at least 1 liter per day per 100 pounds of body weight. This may need to be increased depending on how much you sweat and the climate in which you live.

High Fiber Diet

A diet high in fiber binds organic substances and removes them from the body. Fibers that work well include psyllium husks (one or two tablespoons a day), ground flax seeds (two tablespoons a day), and whole grains.

Glutathione

Glutathione, the liver's strongest antioxidant, helps to purge the body of mercury and other toxins. It is ineffective when taken orally; however, taking 500 mg. of Milk Thistle twice a day or N-Acetyl Cysteine (NAC) 500 to 1000 mg. two to three times a day can help stimulate the liver to produce glutathione.

Supplements Specifically Helpful in Neutralizing Toxins

Supplement	Directions
MSM (Methylsulfonylmethane)	1000 mg. two to three times a day
Vitamin C	Especially Mineral Ascorbates 1000 mg. two or three times a day
B Complex	Once or twice a day to protect the body's enzyme systems
Alpha Lipoic Acid	100 to 200 mg. once or twice a day
Vitamin E	400 to 600 units once a day. (Vitamin E must always be taken with at least 500 to 100 mg. of Vitamin C.)
Selenium	100 to 200 mcgs. once or twice a day

Sweating Heavily

Heavy sweating can be induced actively by exercising or passively by steam baths or sauna, preferably infrared. Sweating is a good way of ridding the body of toxins.

Oral Chelation

Numerous substances act as chelating agents by binding with heavy metals so that they are excreted from the body. What most oral chelators have in common is sulfur. Sulfur is a unique metal that is able to bind to toxins and excrete them from the body in a harmless fashion. Examples include:

Substance	Notes
L-Cysteine	A sulfur-bearing amino acid that facilitates metal detoxification (found in Dandelion and Sarsaparilla). 250 mg—500 mg twice a day
L-Methionine	A sulfur-bearing amino acid that binds with heavy metals (also found in Dandelion and Sarsaparilla).
MSM	A form of sulfur that facilitates metal detoxification. 1,000 mg two-to-three times a day with meals.
Kyolic (odorless garlic)	The sulfur in garlic helps remove mercury from the body.
Cilantro Tincture	Mobilizes mercury out of the tissues.
DMSA (Dimercaptosuccinic Acid)	An oral chelating agent which is very effective in removing most heavy metals.
D-Penicillamine	A medication used for the treatment of rheumatoid arthritis for many years. It is an excellent chelator of all toxic metals. It is taken orally, 250 to 500 mg. three to four times a day twice a week. After six to eight weeks, the urine is reevaluated to see if the job is done. If not, then another round is taken until the urine is clear of heavy metals. Take only under the supervision of an experienced physician, since improper use can result in side effects. D-Penicillamine can be taken with meals, although not simultaneously with vitamins.
Fresh Cilantro	Helps remove heavy metals from the body. Although the stems can be bitter, they may be used in addition to the leaves.

Psyllium Cleanse to Eliminate Toxins through the Bowel

Psyllium absorbs many times its weight in water and works its way through the length of the intestine, forcing out stored wastes that have not been excreted. Bentonite is a clay mixture that also absorbs toxins; however, it can be constipating.

The following psyllium cleanse is taken for five days, three times a day, between meals.

Supplies:
Psyllium seed husks (Yerba Prima, see Resources)
Bentonite liquid (Sonne #7, see Resources)
Shaker bottle with a tight lid (preferably a wide-mouth bottle)
8 ounces of water or juice (apple or cranberry)
8 ounces of extra water

Directions:
1. Add 1 tablespoon of psyllium seed husks to the shaker bottle.
2. Add one quarter cup of Bentonite liquid.
3. Add 8 ounces of water or juice.
4. Shake vigorously and drink immediately.
5. Follow with 8 ounces of water.

During the cleanse, follow your regular diet. When you have finished the cleanse, eat yogurt with active cultures two to three times a day for five days to replenish your bacterial flora. Or you can begin taking Probiotics with each meal.

Water Filters

Reverse osmosis water filters/purifiers are the best option for removing dissolved heavy metals, bacteria, and viruses, as well as other pollutants. Reverse osmosis filters use a semipermeable membrane to remove undesirable substances from water. Polyamide membrane technology is the newest technology in reverse osmosis filtration systems and is available in brands such as Nature's Sunshine (a portable countertop unit) and WaterFactory (an under-the-counter unit).

Many people do not like the taste of reverse osmosis water. In that case, there are some very high-quality filters that will filter out unwanted minerals, as well as bacteria and organic chemicals.

Important Note: When buying bottled water, even distilled or reverse osmosis, one should avoid containers that are opaque or white plastic, and use only clear plastic or glass. If you can taste plastic in the water, the water has plastic in it. With prolonged exposure, plastics have been shown to cause hormonal imbalances that can lead to feminization of men, infertility in women, and impaired brain function.

Removing Metals with Professional Help

Although learning to solve your own health problems is extremely beneficial, you'll need to consult with a doctor or dentist familiar with chemical and metal toxicity if you suspect your body is overwhelmed with metal toxicity.

Replace Your Silver Fillings

Silver fillings are at least one-half mercury and mercury does leach out of the fillings. It is, therefore, critical to have mercury amalgams removed from your teeth. Acceptable substitutes for silver fillings include composite, ceramic, porcelain, and gold. Be sure to use a dentist who is experienced and trained in removal of amalgam fillings, because improper removal can result in increased toxicity and exposure.

The researcher most known for her observations concerning amalgam fillings is Hulda Regehr Clark, Ph.D., N.D. Her books contain extensive information about metal poisoning. Although much of her work contains information for people who are seriously ill with degenerative diseases, the information she's assembled on dental cleanup is useful for anyone who has metal in their mouth. See the Resources section in this chapter for a list of her books.

According to Dr. Frank Jerome, who wrote the Dental Clean-Up section in Hulda Clark's *The Cure for All Diseases,* acceptable plastics include Methyl Methacrylate for dentures (clear only), Flexite for partial dentures (clear only), and Composite Materials for fillings (a material that has been used in front teeth for 30 years).

Intravenous Chelation Therapy

Seriously ill individuals may want to seek the help of a physician who uses intravenous chelation therapy, which works faster than oral chelation. Chelating agents that are used intravenously include:

Substance	Notes
EDTA (Ethylene Diamine Tetraacetic Acid)	A synthetic chelating agent that attracts most toxic metals such as lead, aluminum, mercury, iron, cadmium, and nickel. Vitamins and minerals must be given in conjunction with EDTA so as not to develop a deficiency state.
Intravenous Vitamin C	Followed by intravenous glutathione
Dimercapto-1-propane Sulfonate (DMPS) Mercury Chelation	Also given as suppositories or transdermal applications, DMPS is a chelating agent that is used to remove mercury after amalgam fillings have been removed. DMPS should not be given to patients who have amalgam fillings in their mouth. Suppositories are recommended for children.

Bloodletting

As strange as it may sound, the ancient wisdom of bloodletting did have a basis. There are certain metals and toxins that can best be removed by removing blood on a regular basis. For example, scientists know that men who donate blood decrease their iron levels, which results in a decreased incidence of heart attacks and strokes. Donating blood two or three times a year or even just having blood removed in the form of phlebotomy two to three times a year can be very helpful in decreasing the levels of toxic metals and chemicals.

Chemicals in Food and Personal Products

According to Hulda Clark, the solvent that does the most harm is benzene. This highly carcinogenic molecule has found its way into the water supply because of its heavy use in lawn preparations such as ChemLawn. She has found it in bottled drinking water and fruit juices, including health food store varieties. The next most harmful solvent is isopropyl alcohol (also known as rubbing alcohol). Even in minute amounts, these solvents accumulate in the body and over time will affect the body's nervous system.

The Benefit of Kosher Foods

Interestingly, Hulda found that kosher foods were superior in cleanliness and purity. Kosher canned foods did not have rabbit fluke, sweetened foods did not have asbestos, processed foods did not have azo dye pollution (a parasite), and meats did not have rabbit fluke or ascaris. While the dairy products she tested often had azo dyes, the kosher dairy food was free of parasite eggs.

The Feingold Diet

The Feingold Diet is fastidious in avoiding all kinds of preservatives and additives in food and insists on eating only organically grown food free of insecticides. To avoid the effects of pesticides and other chemicals on fruits and vegetables, you need to use either a fruit and vegetable wash to clean the produce thoroughly, or add a few drops of Clorox to a gallon of water and use that to clean the produce of any residue. Be sure to rinse off well before eating.

Personal Products

Antiperspirants and cosmetics contain aluminum. Talc, a popular ingredient in baby powder, may be contaminated with asbestos. Lipstick and toothpaste both contain metals.

Endocrine Disrupters

Disruptions that occur in the delicately balanced endocrine system are frequently due to drugs that have been inappropriately prescribed, or pollution from industrial chemicals.

Xenobiotics

"Xeno" means foreign or outside of the body. Any substance that is foreign to the body and is not nutritive is a xenobiotic. Xenobiotics are especially common in insecticides and pesticides. Studies over the years have demonstrated that they interfere with hormone production, particularly sperm production in men. If you must be exposed to xenobiotics, especially pesticides and insecticides, wear protective clothing. Always wash fruits and vegetables thoroughly to eliminate insecticides and pesticides. There are fruit and vegetable washes that remove any pesticide residues that are on the surface of produce.

Xenoestrogens

Xenoestrogens are chemicals that confuse the body because they mimic natural estrogens. They cause trauma to human cells and distort the levels of estrogen in the male and female body.

Since the human body cannot distinguish between natural estrogen and xenoestrogens, the xenoestrogens are capable of accumulating within the body and can have a profound estrogen-like impact. They can cause sterilization in men, mood changes, and development of cancer.

Sources of Xenoestrogens

The two biggest sources of xenoestrogens are plastics such as PCB (polychlorinated biphenyls) and pesticides—especially DDT.

Plastics Can Be Toxic
Cloudy and colored plastics tend to leak plastics into the food. Only buy water in glass or clear plastic containers. Microwaving in plastic can cause extreme toxicity. Food microwaved on a plastic surface, whether it is styro-

foam, true plastic, microwavable plastic, or plastic wrap, will cause the food to absorb the plastic at up to 5,000 times the maximum daily exposure allowed by the EPA. Therefore, it is advisable that if you must microwave your food, it should always be done in glass or ceramic containers. **Important Note:** If the food has a plastic taste, it has absorbed the plastic and is toxic to the body.

Toxic Chemicals in the Home

Sources of toxic chemicals in the home include commercial cleaning products, formaldehyde used in paneling and carpeting, and chemicals in paints, floor coatings, and wallpaper. New citrus-based cleaners sold at health food stores offer cleaning solutions that are non-toxic.

If you smell, taste, or are aware of chemicals in your environment, it is best to leave that environment. If that is not possible, see section on Removing Metals: Self Help Measures.

Cleaning Out Your Liver

The liver regulates protein metabolism, secretes bile that is necessary for the digestion of fats, and acts as a detoxifier for the body. Toxins can put a strain on the liver, resulting in digestive disorders, allergies, low energy, and an inability to detoxify harmful substances. N-Acetylcysteine and Silymarin, also known as Milk Thistle, will help the liver produce glutathione, which is the liver's primary means of detoxification.

The Herxheimer Reaction

Detoxification may be accompanied by the Herxheimer Reaction during the first few days or weeks that you detoxify. A release of toxic chemicals from dying bacteria triggers an immune response and may cause flu-like symptoms including nausea, diarrhea and sore throat. Adolf Jerisch, an Australian dermatologist, and

Karl Herxheimer, a German dermatologist, are both credited with the discovery of the condition in 1895.

Coffee Enemas

If you are experiencing a severe Herxheimer Reaction, a coffee enema will help purge toxins from your liver. Coffee taken in the form of an enema goes directly to the liver, where it stimulates production of glutathione but does not cause stimulation of the brain the way it would if you were taking it orally.

Supplies:
Enema bag
Soft rubber colon tube (See Resources)
Spring water
Organic coffee

Directions:
1. Make 2 cups of coffee with organic grounds. Do not use an aluminum coffee maker, as aluminum is a toxic metal. Coffee made the day before is acceptable if you store it in the refrigerator.
2. Fill a pan or jar with one quart of spring water.
3. Add the liquid coffee to the water until the color is a dark amber shade. The temperature should be warm to the touch. Add warm water until you feel that the temperature is right.
4. Fill the enema bag with the coffee mixture you have diluted with water.
5. Find a place to hang your enema bag in your bathroom that is approximately 18-20 inches higher than where you plan to take your enema (e.g. the doorknob if you plan to lie on the floor).
6. Insert the colon tube and release the stopper. It will be difficult to retain the enema at first.
7. Use half of the contents of the enema bag or the entire bag if possible. Try to retain the enema for ten to fifteen minutes.

Note: You will want to clean your enema bag occasionally with water and a tablespoon of Clorox. Clamp off the tube and fill the bag with water. Add one tablespoon of Clorox. Rinse your bag thoroughly after 30 minutes.

Radiation

An often-dismissed form of toxicity in our environment is radiation. More than 8,000 studies have been done worldwide that show how electromagnetic fields affect human health.

Power Lines

Epidemiologist Nancy Wertheimer first uncovered statistics that suggest a link between electromagnetic radiation and cancer in Denver, Colorado in 1980. Although the press has covered this issue for more than twenty years, public health officials have done little to work toward a safe electrical environment. Teachers who work in classrooms near high power lines notice how electromagnetic fields affect children's behavior. They report that children have trouble paying attention, and fidget far more than they do in an area that is not within an electrical field.

Electrical Devices in the Home and at Work

All electrical devices have an electric field that can extend from a few inches to a few feet. Although electromagnetic fields drop off rapidly around the perimeter of an electrical device, one should never sleep close to an electric clock or work next to a copying machine. The ballast transformers at the end of fluorescent lighting fixtures are particularly unhealthy and may cause dizziness for anyone who has built-in electric lighting in their cubicle. Electric blankets, heating pads, and heating elements in water beds are common sources of unhealthy electromagnetic fields. Pregnant women or women who wish to become pregnant are advised not to use electric heating devices.

X-Rays

X-rays are a potent source of radiation. Physicians and chiropractors often order x-rays unnecessarily. Unless your physician or chiropractor is suspecting a serious condition, be sure to ask how taking an x-ray will change the course of treatment. If you are not satisfied with the answer or if you think they are ordering x-rays unnecessarily, get a second opinion. Unnecessary x-rays are a major source of radiation.

In-Flight Radiation from the Sun

Solar radiation is a problem when flying during the day. As a result, it is preferable to fly at night when possible.

Cell Phones

Cell phones emit electromagnetic radiation in the form of radio frequency (RF) radiation. Over the past twenty years, epidemiological groups have studied the effects of the Extremely Low Frequency Band (ELF) of the electromagnetic spectrum at 60 Hz. This is the frequency associated with the electrical lines that supply homes and offices with electrical power. The electromagnetic spectrum is a continuum that is divided into higher and higher frequencies that are used for broadcast equipment and wireless phones.

Although it is assumed that the bands known as RF bands are safe, researchers in Norway and Sweden sent questionnaires to 17,000 people and found that one in four had symptoms such as dizziness, disorientation, nausea, headache, and transient confusion with cell-phone use.

The Electromagnetic Spectrum—How It's Divided and Who's Using It

Just as phones and personal digital assistants are becoming Internet-capable due to advances in wireless technology, so are coffee machines, sprinklers, vending machines, medical devices and air conditioners. The number of devices slated to be controlled through wireless technology may cause us to be immersed in an invisible ocean of electromagnetic radiation. Occupational researchers have not had a chance to study how working with high-frequency bands impact human health.

Band Classification	Frequency	Service
Very Low Frequency (VLF)	Less than 30 Khz	Submarine navigation systems.
Low Frequency (LF)	30 KHz to 300 KHz	Military systems, Ground Wave Emergency Network, beacon stations, European-based broadcasts
Medium Frequency (MF)	300 KHz to 3 MHz	Maritime communications, beacon stations, Travelers Information Service, AM broadcast, cordless telephones, amateur radio, world broadcasting band, standard time and frequency stations, U.S. Coast Guard weather, aircraft communication, short-wave band
High Frequency (HF)	3 MHz to 30 MHz	Short wave band.
Very High Frequency (VHF)	30 MHz to 300 MHz	Television, government, law enforcement, Red Cross, highway maintenance, forestry, utilities, petroleum companies, children's walkie talkies, cordless telephones, amateur radio, pagers, surveillance and eavesdropping equipment, FM broadcast, Civilian Aircraft Weather, police scanners
Ultra High Frequency (UHF)	300 MHz to 3 GHz	Military aircraft band, amateur radio, police, UHF television, mobile business, public safety and mobile satellite radio services, cellular phones
Super High Frequency (SHF)	3 GHz to 30 GHz	Under development by the government and corporations that participated in FCC auctions
Extremely High Frequency	30 GHz to 300 GHz	Under development by the government

Resources

Chelation Therapists

Although the medical establishment does not approve of chelation therapy (despite its safety and efficacy) many people have benefited from the safe removal of metals such as cadmium, lead, and mercury. The American Board of Chelation Therapists certifies doctors in chelation therapy.

The American Board of Chelation Therapy
Establishes required qualifications of licensed physicians, D.O.s, M.D.s for certification as Diplomates in the field of Chelation Therapy, conducts examinations and issues certification as a Diplomate in Chelation Therapy.
1407½ N. Wells Street
Chicago, IL 60610
(312) 787-2228
(800) 356-2228
Email: jackhank@mindspring.com
www.abct.info

Colon Tube, Coffee Enema

Ultra Life carries a soft rubber tube that can be used with any drug-store enema bag. Attach the long rubber tube to the plastic tip that is supplied with the enema bag.

Colon Tube
Ultra Life, Inc.
P.O. Box 440
Carlyle, IL 62232
(618) 594-7711
Email : ullife@accessus.net
www.ultralifeinc.com

Supplies, Psyllium Cleanse

The following products are available in most health food stores.

Sonne No. 7
Bentonite, An absorbent aid in detoxification
Sonne's Organic Foods, Inc.
Kansas City, MO 64142

Psyllium Husks Powder
Yerba Prima, Inc.
740 Jefferson Avenue
Ashland, OR 97520
www.yerba.com

Alliances and Organizations

Alliances and organizations that provide valuable up-to-date information include:

Holistic Dental Association
P.O. Box 5007
Durango, CO 81301
(303) 259-1091

Dental Amalgam Mercury Syndrome, Inc. (DAMS)
025 Osuna Blvd. NE, Suite B
Albuquerque, NM 87109-2523
(505) 888-0111

Citizens for Health
5 Thomas Circle NW, Suite 500
Washington, DC 20005
Telephone: (202) 483-4344
Fax: (202) 462-6534
Web Site: www.citizens.org
Contact: Ana Micka, President & CEO, amicka@citizens.org

Dr. Clark Research Organization
David P. Amrein, based in Switzerland, is president of the Dr. Clark Research
Association. He has created a Web site at www. drclark. net and writes a monthly
newsletter that is available in print and e-mail formats.

Holistic Dental Association
P.O. Box 5007
Durango, CO 81301
(303) 259-1091

Water Filtration Systems

Nature's Sunshine and WaterFactory reverse-osmosis water filters are available from the following dealers:

Enviro Health Environmental Home Inspections, Inc.
7104 Red Top Road
Hummelstown, PA 17036
Telephone: (717) 583-4155 or (888) 735-9649
Fax: (717) 583-0536
Email: envirohomeinfo@mindspring.com
www.create-your-healthy-home.com
Contact: May E. Dooley

Doctor's Data
3755 Illinois Avenue
St. Charles, IL 60174-2420
(800) 323-2784
www.doctorsdata.com

Great Smokies Laboratory
63 Zillicoa Street
Asheville, NC 28801-1074
(800) 522-4762
www.gsdl.com

CHAPTER 11

I hope that *Brain Fog* has widened your perspective concerning the different causes, possible treatments, and the various avenues of healing that you can pursue when dealing with a lack of mental clarity. Obviously, *Brain Fog* is not a medical text upon which to rely for diagnosis and treatment. If you have taken care of the basics, for example getting adequate sleep, exercising regularly, drinking enough water (enough means urine turns clear), and eating a high quality healthy diet and you still do not feel as good as you could, you will need the assistance of a physician who can outline a program of detoxification, appropriately checking you for hypoglycemia, thyroid conditions, hormone and immune status, rule out more serious conditions such as heart disease, diabetes, and cancer, and evaluate whether you have any nutritional deficiencies. Do not hesitate to find a physician who is knowledgeable and open minded about pursuing whatever avenue you need to heal. To quote the *Ethics of the Fathers*, "If someone said he tried and did not succeed, do not believe him. If someone says he didn't try but did succeed, do not believe him. If someone said he tried and succeeded, believe him." In other words, do not give up until you find the solution to your problem. It may take time, money, and effort but you are worth it!

There is one more important thing that I would like to address—perhaps *the* most important thing—which is the discussion of the Spirit. Call it the soul, spirit, Higher Power, or G-d—we are all talking about that which makes life meaningful. Being connected with our Creator and acknowledging that there is a Higher Power who intimately cares about each and every one of us infuses our life with purpose and joy. Having a close relationship with our Higher Power and knowing that everything G-d sends us is for our benefit, growth and higher good—even though it may not be apparent at the time—allows us to relax and enjoy the journey, rather than fretting that we have not reached a certain self-conceived destination. As fellow travelers in this journey, we must learn to treat love as a verb and look forward to giving. The universe is not random. Everything is Divine Providence.

Search for the blessings in all things and all things will be a blessing. I leave you with the traditional Jewish blessing "L'Chaim! —To life!"

About the Author

Binyamin Rothstein, D.O.

Dr. Binyamin Rothstein has been in private practice in Baltimore, Maryland since 1986. He attended medical school at Des Moines University College of Osteopathic Medicine and served three years in the United States Army at the United States Army Medical Research Institute of Infectious Diseases. In addition to being board certified in Family Practice, he is also a Diplomate of the American Board of Chelation Therapy and has been awarded certificates of competency in Cranial Osteopathy. He is a Diplomate of the American Board of Anti-Aging Medicine and is also an adjunct clinical assistant professor of Osteopathic Manipulative Medicine and of Family Practice at the New York College of Osteopathic Medicine.

Dr. Rothstein has conducted workshops on the treatment of children with ADHD, and lectured on Brain Fog and Nutritional Medicine, as well as chronic and acute pain conditions. He has authored articles on back pain and back injuries and has also lectured on the treatment of heart disease using chelation therapy. Dr. Rothstein has developed special expertise in hormone replacement therapies, detoxification, ADHD, and sports injuries. He is a member of the American College for Advancement in Medicine, the American Academy of Anti-Aging Medicine, the Baltimore County Medical Society, the Cranial Academy, the American Academy of Osteopathy, the American Osteopathic Association, and the Maryland Association of Osteopathic Physicians. Dr. Rothstein resides with his wife and eight children in Baltimore and enjoys hiking, bicycle riding, studying Chasidic philosophy, and mentoring young adults.

Dr. Rothstein can be contacted at his private office in Baltimore, Maryland at (410) 484-2121 or you can visit him on the web at www.docben.com.

What is a D.O.?

D.O. is an abbreviation for Doctor of Osteopathy. In the United States, D.O.s and allopathic physicians (M.D.s) are the only physicians fully trained and licensed to prescribe medicine and perform surgery. Both groups practice and specialize in all branches of medicine and surgery. To a D.O., however, you are more than just a collection of body parts. Osteopathic physicians concentrate on treating your body as a whole, because they understand how all the body's systems are interconnected and how each one affects the other.

Osteopathic physicians specializing in osteopathic manipulative techniques focus special attention on the musculoskeletal system and use their hands to identify and treat structural problems, supporting the body's natural tendency toward health and healing. This additional training allows a D.O. to care effectively for patients and relieve their distress, oftentimes without the need for drugs and surgery. If you would like to see an osteopathic physician, the following organizations can help you find a doctor in your area:

The Cranial Academy
8202 Clearvista Pkwy. #9-D
Indianaoplis, IN 46256
(317) 594-0411
www.cranialacademy.org

American Academy of Osteopathy
3500 DePauw Blvd, Ste. 1080
Indianapolis, IN 46268
(317) 879-1881
Fax (317) 879-0563
www.academyofosteopathy.org

BIBLIOGRAPHY

Chapter 3—Stress and Fatigue

Arnsten, A. The Biology of Being Frazzled. Science. 12 June 1998; 280:1711-12.

Scott, L., Dinan, T. The Neuroendocrinology of Chronic Fatigue Syndrome: Focus on the Hypothalamic-Pituitary-Adrenal Axis. Functional Neurology 1999; 14:3-11.

Chrousos, G. P. The Role of Stress and the Hypothalamic-Pituitary-Adrenal Axis in the Pathogenesis of the Metabolic Syndrome: Neuro-endocrine and target tissue-related causes. Intl. J of Obesity 2000; 24.

Ron de Kloet, E., Oitzl, M., Joels, M. Stress and Cognition: Are Corticosteroids Good or Bad Guys? Trends Neurosci 1999; 22:422-426.

Tilders, F.J.H., Schmidt, E.D., Hoogedijk, W.J.G., Swaab, D.F. Delayed Effects of Stress and Immune Activation. Bailliere's Cl Endo and Metab. 1999: Vol 13 No 4; 523-540.

Martin, S., Wraith, P., Deary, I., and Douglas, N. The Effect of Nonvisable Sleep Fragmentation on Daytime Function. A.M. J R Respir Crit Care Med 1997; 155:1596-1601.

Sapolsky, R. Glucocorticoids, Stress, and Their Adverse Neurological Effects: Relevance to Aging. Exper Geron. 1999; 34:721-732.

Vaidya, V., J Biosci. 2000; Vol 25 No 2: 123-124.

Pusciglio, J. et al. Stress, Aging, and Neurodegenerative Disorders.

O'Connor, T.M., O'Halloran, D.J., Shanahan, F. The Stress Response and the Hypothalamic Pituitary Adrenal Axis: From Molecule to Melancholia. Q J Med. 2000; 93:323-333.

Chapter 4—Hypothyroidism

Caselli, R.J., Graff-Radford N.R., Reimanem, Weaver A., Osborne, B., Lucas, J., Uecker, A., Thibodeau, S.N., <u>Preclinical Memory Decline in Cognitively Normal Apolipoprotein e-4 Homozygotes</u>. Neurology 1999; 53:201-207.

Braunwald et al., <u>Harrison's Principles of Internal Medicine.</u> 15 Edition, McGraw-Hill, 2001.

Wilson et al. <u>Williams Textbook of Endocrinology 9th Edition</u> 1998 W.B. Saunders Company.

Hardman, J.G. and Limbird, L.E. <u>Goodman and Gilman's: The Pharmacological Basis of Therapeutics 9th Edition</u> 1996.

Chapter 5—Sex Hormones

Cutler, W., Genovese-Stone, E. <u>Disease a Month: Wellness in Women After 40 Years of Age: The Role of Sex Hormones and Pheromones</u>. September 1998 Vol 44 No 9.

Seidman, S., Walsh, B. <u>Testosterone and Depression in Aging Men</u>. Am J Geriatr Psychiatry 7:1, Winter 1999.

Slater, S. and Oliver, R.T.D. <u>Testosterone: Its Role in Development of Prostate Cancer and Potential Risk from Use as Hormone Replacement Therapy</u>. Drugs and Aging 2000 December 17 (6) 431-439.

Grinspoon, S. et al. <u>The Effects of Hypogonadism and Testosterone Administration of Depression Indices in HIV-Infected Men</u>. J of C Endo Crin and Metab 2000 Volume 85 No 1 (60—65).

Simon, J. <u>Safety of Estrogen/Androgen Regiments</u>. J of Reprod Med March 2001 Vol 45 No 3 (281-290).

Rolf, C., Nieschlaj, E. <u>Potential Adverse Effects of Long-Term Testosterone Therapy</u> Bailliere's Clin Endo and Metab October 1998 Vol 12 No 3 (521-534).

Davis, S.R. <u>The Therapeutics of Androgens in Women</u>. J of Steroid Bio Chem and Mol Biol: 1999; 69 (177-184).

English, K. et al <u>Low-Dose Transdermal Testosterone Therapy Improves Angina Threshold in Men with Chronic Stable Angina</u>. Circulation. 2000; 102:1906-1911.

Rhoden, E.L., Morgentaler, A. <u>Testosterone Replacement Therapy in Hypogonadal Men at High Risk for Prostate Cancer: Results of One Year of Treatment in Men with Prostatic Intraepithelial Neoplasia</u>. December 2003; 170:2348-2351.

Graziottin, L. <u>Libido: The Biologic Scenario</u>. Maturitas. 2000: 34; S1–S1 6.

Huppert, F.A., Van Niekerk, J.K. <u>Dehydroepiandrosterone (DHEA) Supplementation for Cognitive Function.</u> Chocrane Database of Systematic Views 2002 Issue 1 (1 to 19).

Morales, A.J. et al <u>Effects of Replacement Dose of Dehydroepiandrosterone in Men and Women of the Advancing Age</u>. J of Clin Endocrin and Metab 1994: 78, 6 (1360-1367).

Sherwin, B. <u>Estrogen and Cognitive Functioning in Women.</u> Estrogen and Cognition 1999; 217(17-22).

Toren, P., Dor, J., Rehavim, Weizman, A. <u>Hypothalamic-Pituitary-Ovarian Axis and Mood</u>. Biol Psych: 1996; 40; 1050-1055.

Small, G. <u>Estrogen Effects on the Brain</u>. The Journal of Gender-Specific Med 1998; 1 (2:23-27).

Van Amelsvoort, T., Compton, J., and Murphy, D. <u>*In Vivo* Assessment of Estrogen on the Human Brain.</u> Trends in Endo and Metabo. August 2001; 12:6 (273-276).

Fink, G. et al <u>Estrogen Control of Central Neurotransmission: Throughout the Mood, Mental State, and Memory</u>. Cell and Molec Neurobio 1996; 16:3 (325-344).

Wise, P. et al <u>Estrogens: Trophic and Protective Factors in the Adult Brain</u>. Frontiers in Neuroendocr. 2001; 22:33-66.

Harden, C. The Mysterious Effect of Reproductive Hormones on Cognitive Function: Scientific Knowledge in Search of an Application. JGSM October 2000 33-37.

Genazzani, A.R. et al Menopause and Essential Nervous System: Intervention Options. Maturitas 1999; 31:103-110.

McEwen, B.S. Steroid Hormones: Effect on Brain Development and Function. Horm Res 1992; 37 (Suppl 3): 1-10.

Majewska, M.B. Neurosteroids: Endogenous Bimodal Modulators of the GABA a Receptor. The Mechanism of Action and Physiological Significance. Progr in Neurobio 1992; 38:379-395.

Fillith, Luine, V. The Neurobiology of Gonadal Hormones and Cognitive Decline in Late Life. Meturitas. 1997; 26:159-164.

Chapter 6—Hypoglycemia

Felig et al, Endocrinology and Metabolism Third Edition; McGraw Hill, Incorporated: 1995:776-8, 1251-67, 1761-64.

Chapter 7—Food Allergies

Chapter 8—Important Nutrients and Common Nutritional Deficiencies

Shils et al, Modern Nutrition in Health and Disease, Ninth Edition, Williams and Williams, 1994.

Textbook of Biochemistry, Fourth Edition, Devlin et al, Wiley-Less 1997.

Heller et al. Lipid Mediators in Inflammatory Disorders. Drugs, April 1998; 55 (4):47-96.

Scientific American Medicine 2003 Volume 4 Chapter 13: 14-16.

Smith, D.L. et al <u>Eskimo Plasma Constituents, Dihomo-Gama Linolenic Acid, Eicosapentaenoic Acid, and Docosahexaenoic Acid Inhbiit the Release of Atherogenic Mitogens, Lipids,</u> Volume 24 #1 (1989):70-75.

Belch, J.J., Hill, A. <u>Evening Primrose Oil and Borage Oil in Rheumatologic Conditions.</u> A.J. of Clin Nutr. 71 (1 Suppl):352S-6S, 2000 Jan.

Kenny, F.S. et al. <u>Gamma Linolenic Acid with Tamoxifen as Primary Therapy in Breast Cancer.</u> Intl J of C. 85 (5):643-8, 2000 March 1.

Lang, G.C. et al. <u>Essential Fatty Acids and Cardiovascular Disease: The Edinburgh Artery Study.</u> Vasc Med. 4 (4): 219-26, 1999.

Goh, Y.K. et al. <u>The Effect of Omega 3 Fatty Acid on Plasma Lipids, Cholesterol and Lipo Protein Fatty Acid Content in NIDDM Patients.</u> Diabetologia. 40 (1):45-52, 1997 Jan.

Mohan, I.K, Das, U.N. <u>Oxidant Stress, Antioxidants, and Essential Fatty Acids in Systemic Lupus Erythematosus.</u> Prostaglandins Leukotrienes and Essential Fatty Acids. 56 (3): 193-8, 1997 March.

Ghosh, J., Myers, Jr. C.E., <u>Arachidonic Acid Metabolism and Cancer of the Prostate.</u> Nutrition 14: 48-57, 1998.

Uauy, R., Mena, P., Rojas, C. <u>Essential Fatty Acids in Early Life: Structural and Functional Role.</u> Proc of the Nutr Soc (2000), 59:3-15.

Youdim, K.A., Martin, A., Joseph, J.A. <u>Essential Fatty Acids and the Brain: Possible Health Implications.</u> Int. J. Devl Neurosci 18 (2000): 383-399.

Chapter 9—Infectious Diseases

Caselli, R.J. et al. <u>Preclinicial Memory Decline in Cognitively Normal Apo Lipo Protein e-4 Homozygotes.</u> Neurology 1999; 53:201-207.

Stratton, C.W., Mitchell, W.M., Sriram, S. <u>Editorial: Does Chlamydia *Pneumoniae* Play a Role in the Pathogenesis of Multiple Sclerosis?</u> J. Med. Microbiol. Volume 49 (2000), 1-3.

Lin, W.R., Casas, I., Wilicock, G.K, Itzhaki, R.F. Neurotropic Viruses and Alzheimer's Disease: A Search for Varicella Zoster Virus DNA by the Polymerase Chain Reaction. J. Neurol. Neurosurg Psych 1997; 62:586-89.

Stephenson, J. New Studies Illuminate Brain Disorders. JAMA, February 10, 1999, Volume 281; 6: 499-501.

Greenlee, J.E., Rose, J.W. Controversies in Neurological Infectious Diseases. Sem. In Neurol. 20 (3):375-76, 2000.

Braunwald et al., Harrison's Principles of Internal Medicine. 15 Edition, McGraw-Hill, 2001.

Chapter 10—Toxicity

Rojan, W., Ware, J. Exposure to Lead in Children—How Low is Low Enough. N Engl J Med April 2003. 348; 16; 1515-1516.

Canfield, R. et al Intellectual Impairment in Children With Blood Lead Concentrations Below 10 ug per Deciliter. N Engl J of Med. April 2003. 348;16:1517-26.

Fitzgerald, W., Clarkson, T. Mercury and Monomethylmercury: Present and Future Concerns. Environmental Health Perspectives 1991; 96:159-166.

Bluhm, R. et al Elemental Mercury Vapor Toxicity, Treatment, and Prognosis After Acute, Intensive Exposure in Chloralkali Plant Workers. Part 1: History, Neuropsychological Findings and Chelators Effects. Human and Experim Toxic. 1992; 11:201-210.

Herada, M. et al Methylmercury Level in Umbilical Cords from Patients with Congenital Minamata Disease. Sci of the Total Environ. 1999; 234:59-62.

Eto, K. et al. The Differential Diagnosis Between Organic and Inorganic Mercury Poisoning In Human Cases—The Pathologic Point of View. Toxicol Path. 1999; 27, 6:664-671.

O'Connor, N. The Toxicity of Mercury—Myth or Reality?

Siblerud, R. <u>The Relationship Between Mercury from Dental Amalgam and Mental Health.</u> Amer J of Psychoth October 1989; 43, 4:575-587.

Hanson, M. and Pleva, J. <u>The Dental Amalgam Issue. A Review</u>. 1991 Experientia; 47: 9-22.

Hardman, J.G. and Limbird, L.E. <u>Goodman and Gilman's: The Pharmacological Basis of Therapeutics 9—Edition</u> 1996.

Fitzgerald, W.F., Clarkson, T.W. <u>Mercury and Monomethyl Mercury: Present and Future Concerns</u>. Environ Healt Persp Volume 96, 1991: 159-166.

Bluhm, R.E. et al. <u>Elemental Mercury Vapor Toxicity, Treatment, and Prognosis After Acute Intensive Exposure in Chloralkali Plant Workers.</u> Part 1: History, Neuropsychological Findings and Chelator Effects. Human and Experi Tox (1992), 11: 201-210.

Harada, M. and Akagi, H. et al. <u>Methylmercury Level in Umbilical Cords from Patients with Congenital Minamata Disease.</u> The Sci of the Tot Environ 234 (1999): 59-62.

Eto, K., Takizawa, Y. et al. <u>Differential Diagnosis Between Organic and Inorganic Mercury Poisoning in Human Cases—The Pathologic Point of View.</u> Toxic Path 1999, 27; 6:664-671

O'Connor, N. <u>The Toxicity of Mercury—Myth or Realty</u>

Siblerud, R.L. <u>The Relationship Between Mercury from Dental Amalgam and Mental Health. A</u>mer J of Psychoth October 1989 (43); 4:576-587.

Hanson, M., Bleva, J. <u>The Dental Amalgam Issue. A Review.</u> Experientia 47 (1991): 9-22.

Choi, B.H. <u>The Effects of Methyl Mercury on the Developing Brain.</u> Progress in Neurobio 1989; 32:447-470.

<u>Intellectual Impairment in Children With Blood Lead Concentrations Below 10 ug per Deciliter</u>, Canfield et al, Volume 348, #16, April 17, 2003, page 1517-1526.

APPENDIX A

World's Best Chicken Soup

(Don't Argue with a Jewish Mother)

Equipment and Ingredients
1 large pot (at least 8 quarts)
1 whole quartered kosher chicken (kosher chicken makes a difference—skin it if you want, but it is not necessary, just take off any feathers)
8 whole carrots, peel but do not cut (add more if you love carrots)
1 whole parsnip, peel but do not cut
1 whole onion, peel but do not cut
3 whole stalks of celery—do not cut
1 entire bulb of fresh garlic, diced
2 bay leaves
1 bunch of fresh dill
4 teaspoons salt (or to taste)
2 dashes white pepper

Directions:
Put the chicken pieces in the pot. Cover with cold water. Bring to a boil. Skim off the "sham," the grayish white foam that comes up when it comes to a boil. **Important Note:** Do not skip this step—it is crucial. Do not add any vegetables or spices until you skim the sham! After the sham has been skimmed, put in the vegetables and spices. Cook covered on a low boil for 1-1/2 to 2 hours. Enjoy!

APPENDIX B

Products

The following products are helpful in optimizing brain function, reducing brain fog, and enhancing your overall health. Although this list is quite comprehensive, it is by no means an exhaustive list of all possible products and compounds that can benefit brain function. The products listed here are ones that I have found particularly useful.

Alpha Lipoic Acid

This antioxidant enhances brain function by alleviating and in some cases reversing the damage caused by free radicals. Taken intravenously or orally, it is beneficial in treating diabetics with diabetic peripheral neuropathy and people with coronary artery disease. The racemic form of Alpha Lipoic Acid has been shown to be five to ten times more potent than its parent compound. The usual dose of Lipoic Acid is 100 to 200 mg. The racemic form is 20 to 30 mg. Alpha Lipoic Acid is extremely safe and nontoxic even when taken at high doses.

CoQ10 (Coenzyme Q10)

Both a free radical scavenger and antioxidant, CoQ10 enhances function of the mitochondria (the powerhouse of the cells) and is instrumental in the repair of cellular membranes. The usual dose is 60 to 240 mg. a day and is best taken with meals in which there is some fat. Newer forms of CoQ10, such as Q Gel, require lower doses because of apparently improved absorption. It is an expensive supplement, so test your CoQ10 levels first to see if you really need it.

Deprenyl (i.e. Eldepryl)

Deprenyl is an MAO B inhibitor that has been shown to improve memory and which also acts as an antidepressant. Since its function is confined to the brain, you do not need to take the precautions that are necessary with the typical MAO inhibitors. Typical dosage is 5 to 10 mg. a day.

DHEA (Dehydroepiandrosterone)

For both men and women, DHEA enhances mood, memory, and immune system functioning (i.e., it increases resistance to disease, including cancer). Women have an additional benefit of being able to convert DHEA into testosterone. DHEA should be supplemented only under the care of a qualified health practitioner. Dosages for men are typically 25 to 50 mg. with supper, and for women as low as 5 to 10 mg. with supper (but some women may need more).

DMSA (Dimercapto Succinic Acid, also known as Succimer)

DMSA is an oral chelating agent that removes mercury and other toxic metals from the body by attaching itself to those toxic metals and thus enabling them to be excreted through the kidneys. It is an effective treatment for heavy metal toxicity and poisoning from substances such as mercury, lead, arsenic, cadmium, nickel, and aluminum. I typically use 500 mg. three times a week for five weeks and then recheck the urine for heavy metals.

Dopamine

For those individuals who are deficient in Dopamine and are experiencing effects such as ADD and ADHD, medications (see list of medications below) may offer the best means of treating that condition. Some people self-medicate with caffeine and nicotine, which can obviously impact their health in a negative manner. Other means of increasing brain levels of Dopamine include intense exercise and L-Tyrosine.

Medications include: Adderall, Ritalin, Cylert, Provigil, Methylin, Metadate, Strattera, Concerta, and Dexedrine.

D-Penicillamine

D-Penicillamine is a drug used for the treatment of rheumatoid arthritis. It is an excellent chelator of heavy metals, including iron, lead, mercury, copper, aluminum, cobalt, and arsenic. Its use should be directed by a physician qualified in prescribing Penicillamine. The typical dose is 500 mg. three to four times a day, two days a week. Typically at that dose, complications and side effects are rare.

EDTA (Ethylene Diamine Tetraacetic Acid)

EDTA is a chelator of divalent cations such as iron, lead, mercury, copper, and aluminum. It has been used intravenously for over 40 years for the treatment of heart disease and strokes. Most recently, it is available as an oral or rectal suppository. Despite its effectiveness and safety, the conventional medical establishment prefers dangerous but lucrative procedures such as bypass surgery.

5-HTP (Five-Hydroxy Tryptophan)

5-Hydroxy Tryptophan (5-HTP) is a precursor to serotonin that easily crosses the blood brain barrier. 5-HTP elevates mood, controls food cravings, serves as an antidepressant, enhances sleep quality, and helps with insomnia. I have found that 5-HTP is beneficial for people who wake in the middle of the night and have a hard time falling back to sleep. An effective dose is between 50 and 300 mg. at bedtime.

Galantamine

Galantamine is an acetylcholinesterase inhibitor that enhances brain function in people suffering from senility, Alzheimer's, or brain fog. It prolongs the effect of the neurotransmitter acetylcholine in the brain by blocking its breakdown by acetylcholinesterase. Galantamine improves the function of the brain, keeping more of the neurotransmitters active. The dose is usually 8 mg. three times a day for a maximum of 24 mg. a day. This is a very potent treatment; therefore, you should start with 8 mg. once a day and gradually build up to the full dose.

Gerovital H3 (GH3)

GH3 is a Procaine compound that was discovered by Dr. Anna Aslan, a physician in Bucharest, Romania. Its use as an anti-aging agent seems to stem from modulating the effect that stress has on the nervous system. It has antidepressant effects, is not addicting, and side effects are minimal. I have found it to be one of the best products for the treatment of stress-related conditions and for anxiety disorders. It can be taken orally twice a day on an empty stomach—25 days on and 5 days off. This can be continued indefinitely. It can also be taken by injection 3 to 5 ccs. given intramuscularly three times a week for one month and then with a break for one to four weeks followed by a repeat of the injections. Many people begin with the injections and then go on to the pills, taking the injections only as needed, if at all. This is an excellent product and although it is over-the-counter, it should be taken only under the guidance of a physician familiar with the product.

Glutathione (GSH)

Glutathione (GSH) is the body's most potent antioxidant. Produced primarily in the liver and the brain, it is critical for preventing damage by toxins and infections. It is a crucial ingredient for the liver to detoxify itself and the blood and for stabilizing the nerve cells in the brain. It is enhanced by taking Milk Thistle (Silymarin) and/or N-Acetyl Cysteine (NAC). GSH is best taken intravenously. Oral preparations are usually ineffective unless they are in the "reduced" form and even then, much is lost during the digestive process.

Huperzine

Huperzine is an acetylcholinesterase inhibitor that is less potent but also much less expensive than Galantamine. It enhances memory and helps reverse the effects of Alzheimer's. The typical dose is 50 mg. twice a day and is best taken on an empty stomach.

L-Glutamine

L-Glutamine enhances bowel function, brain function, muscle tone, endurance, and the production of growth hormone. Typically it is taken 2000 mg. at bedtime and 1000 mg. in the morning upon awakening. It is always best taken on an empty stomach.

L-Tyrosine

L-Tyrosine is necessary for production of the thyroid hormone, as well as for production of Serotonin in the brain. The typical dose is 1000 mg. twice a day.

Milk Thistle (also known as Silymarin)

Milk thistle stimulates production of Glutathione in the liver. In the liver, Milk thistle enhances detoxification of the liver from infection or toxins. The typical dose is 250 to 500 mg. twice a day.

MSM (Methyl Sulfonyl Methane)

MSM (Methyl Sulfonyl Methane) is an excellent source of sulfur. MSM enhances brain function, brain repair and immune function. It also calms the inflammatory response, improves joint function, and helps treat arthritis. It is extremely safe and well tolerated. The usual dose is 1000 to 2000 mg. twice a day with or without food.

NAC (N-Acetyl Cysteine)

NAC (N-Acetyl Cysteine) stimulates production of Glutathione in the liver, thereby enhancing the liver's ability to detoxify the blood. This helps alleviate the brain of its burden of toxins. It also loosens thick mucous in the lungs commonly found with bronchitis and smoker's cough. The typical dose is 250 to 500 mg. twice a day. (For bronchitis, 500 to 1000 mg. twice a day.)

Phosphatidyl Serine

100 to 200 mg. of Phosphatidyl Serine once a day has been shown to improve brain function, enhance memory, recall, and learning skills, even in younger populations.

Pregnenolone

Pregnenolone is a precursor to progesterone utilized by the brain to enhance memory. It also induces sleep at doses as low as 30 mg. to as high as 200 mg. and is beneficial for people who have had a concussion.

Seraphos

Not to be confused with Phosphatidyl Serine, Seraphos is a combination of phosphorus and serine that modulates the effect of cortisol on the brain. Seraphos is very helpful for people suffering from concussions as well as head trauma and who have had or are presently undergoing a great deal of stress. The typical dose is one capsule twice a day.

Serotonin

Serotonin has two areas of primary function: the bowels and the brain. Serotonin is a neurotransmitter and an antidepressant, and improves brain function. It is responsible for keeping the mood elevated and enhancing sleep quality. It generally makes life more fun.

Tryptophan

Tryptophan is a precursor of serotonin; therefore, it is an antidepressant that also enhances brain function and elevates the mood. It is a very safe supplement; although questions were raised by a contaminated batch from Japan that caused a condition known as Eosinophilia-Myalgia Syndrome. For this reason, Tryptophan products were taken off of the market in 1990 but are now available over the counter. The typical dose is 500 to 1000 mg. twice a day.

Vitamin C (Ascorbic Acid)

Vitamin C is an excellent free radical scavenger that helps prevent the effects of free radicals on the body, such as the breakdown of tissues. It is important for the repair of any cell and provides an enhanced response to stress. Volumes have been written about its use in chronic diseases, cancer, infections and arthritis, and in enhancing brain function. The minimum effective dose for adults is 500 mg. twice a day, but Linus Pauling, Ph.D., recommended doses as high as 10 grams twice a day. Some suggest combining it with minerals to form a mineral ascorbate or calcium ascorbate which enhances its availability and decreases such side effects as diarrhea. It can also be given intravenously as high as 100 grams (100,000 mg.)

Vitamin D

Vitamin D is a hormone produced by the skin in reaction to sunlight. It elevates the mood, improves response to stress, and is also necessary for the absorption of calcium. For this reason, it is helpful for the treatment and prevention of osteoporosis. It may be a critical factor in Seasonal Affective Disorder (SAD). The typical dose is 400 to 1000 units a day.

Vitamin E (Alpha-Tocopherol)

Vitamin E is an excellent free radical scavenger that must be taken with vitamin C. It has been shown to be beneficial in patients with Alzheimer's Disease, heart disease, or fatigue syndrome, and can enhance endurance in competitive athletes. The D Alpha-Tocopherol form is the effective form of vitamin E, whereas the L form has been shown not only to be ineffective but also may block the effectiveness of the D form. A typical dose is 400 to 600 units a day with vitamin C 500 mg. twice a day. Larger doses do not seem to confer any additional benefit.

INDEX

Q

978-0-595-33894-8
0-595-33894-1

Printed in the United States
52668LVS00004B/370-441

9 780595 338948